2003

Royal College of Paediatrics and Child Health

PATRON
HRH The Princess Royal

RCPCH

BPA • 75 Years of Service to Children • RCPCH

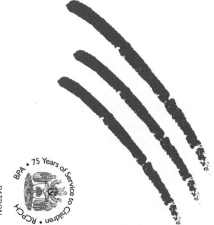

Neonatal and Paediatric Pharmacists Group

Published by RCPCH Publications Limited
50 Hallam Street, London W1W 6DE
Tel: 020 7307 5600
Fax: 020 7307 5601

© 2003 RCPCH Publications Limited

ISBN 190095469 9

Produced by Chamberlain Dunn Associates,
Gothic House, 3 The Green, Richmond TW9 1PL
Tel: 020 8334 4500
Fax: 020 8332 7201
email: mail@chamberdunn.co.uk
website: www.chamberlaindunn.com

Printed by Garda, Essex, UK

Copies may be obtained direct from:

Direct Books,
PO Box 4995,
Poole,
Dorset BH12 3WF
Tel: 01202 712937
Fax: 01202 712930
email: rcpch@bebc.co.uk
web: www.directbooks.uk.com

Not for sale in the United States of America
or Canada

Notice

Pocket Medicines for Children is an
independently written publication designed as a
guide to those who prescribe and dispense
medicines for children. Out of date copies should
not be used. The contributors, reviewers, editorial
board, publishers and printers cannot accept
liability for any errors or omissions.

Every effort has been made to ensure that the
contents herein are accurate and in accord with
the standards accepted at the time of publication.
As new research and experience broaden our
knowledge, changes in treatment and drug
therapy occur. The reader is advised to check the
product information sheet (if available) included
in the package of each product he or she plans to
prescribe or dispense. This is of particular
importance for new or infrequently used
products. The use of unlicensed medicines and of
licensed medicines for unlicensed applications is
explained on pages xvi to xviii of *Medicines for
Children*. Those who prescribe or dispense
remain responsible for what they are doing.

iii | Contents

Preface	*iv*
Introductory notes	*v*
Glossary of terms	*vii*
Abbreviations	*viii*
Symbols	*viii*
Adverse reactions	*x*
Life support (initial management)	*ix*
Weight and body surface area	*xiii*
Monographs	*1*
Nutrition Tables	*315*
Index	*319*

The second edition of *Pocket Medicines for Children* comes 2 years after its first publication which proved to be a popular and practical formulary, particularly for the junior doctor on call. The new edition is required to reflect changes in paediatric practice. It complements the recently published second edition of *Medicines for Children* to which readers should refer for more comprehensive advice and guidance.

The information in *Pocket Medicines for Children* relies entirely on the enormous amount of work put into the second edition of *Medicines for Children* by a large number of contributors and reviewers. Their assistance is appreciated and gratefully acknowledged. The responsibility of collating this information once again fell to Anne Burns whose energy and experience ensured the efficient production of this highly valued formulary.

The Editorial Board is grateful for comments and encouragement from readers to help guide future development of this publication.

Dennis Carson
Chair of the Editorial Board

DRUG MONOGRAPHS

The drug monographs are presented in alphabetical order by generic name and are indexed. Most of the preparations are only listed with the generic name but occasionally a trade name is also given for clarity. In most cases dosage information is presented in tabular form as in *Medicines for Children*. The doses are generally stated on a specific dose per weight basis or by an age/weight range. Occasionally they are stated on a specific dose/surface area basis.

Route	Age				Frequency (times daily)	Notes
	birth–1 month	1 month–2 years	2–12 years	12–18 years		
Oral	1mg/kg	← 2mg/kg →		20mg	4	
IV bolus	← 300–400 microgram/kg →			10–15mg	single dose	

Wherever possible, to avoid confusion and errors, doses have been expressed in whole numbers of units, for example 100 microgram not 0.1mg, 100 nanogram not 0.1 microgram. For reference, 1kg = 1000g, 1g = 1000mg, 1mg = 1000 microgram, 1 microgram = 1000 nanogram.

An example of a monograph table is given. The actual dose to be prescribed/administered is stated in the shaded part of the table followed by the frequency of dosing in a separate column. This method is chosen in preference to stating the total daily dose which requires further calculation to derive the actual dose to be prescribed/administered. Occasionally, if appropriate, a maximum total daily dose is given for some medications in the 'Notes' column. A small number of tables will state a dose to be prescribed/administered on the basis of both weight and age within the same age band e.g. clonazepam. The table on page vi shows how this is clearly marked with a warning to avoid a dosage error.

Route	Age				Frequency (times daily)	Notes
	birth–1 month	1 month–2 years	2–12 years	12–18 years		
Oral	–	**DOSE BY WEIGHT** ◄— 25 microgram/kg —►		–	1	<u>Starting dose.</u> May be given at night.
		DOSE BY AGE <u>≤5 years</u> 250 microgram		1mg	1	Higher, divided doses have been used (up to 100 microgram/kg/**day**).
		<u>5–12 years</u> 500 microgram			1	

USE OF RECOMMENDED INTERNATIONAL NON-PROPRIETARY NAMES (rINN) AND BRITISH APPROVED NAMES (BAN).

Directive 92/27EEC requires use of the rINN for medicinal substances. In the majority of cases the BAN and rINN were identical. Where the two differ, the BAN has been modified to accord with the rINN. In Pocket Medicines for Children the rINN has been used for these medicines with the BAN stated in brackets, for example furosemide (frusemide). The only exception is for adrenaline where preference will continue to be given to the BAN and the name will appear as adrenaline (epinephrine).

GLOSSARY OF TERMS

'Specials'

Medicinal products in respect of which a Product Licence is not in existence but which have been made by the holder of a special manufacturer's licence to the order of a practitioner for administration to a particular patient. Practitioners who order 'specials' should be aware that they have a responsibility for the safety and efficacy of that product for their particular patient. Pharmacists who procure and sell on or supply 'specials' have a responsibility for the inherent quality and safety of the product being sold or supplied.

Extemporaneously prepared medicinal products

These are products which are prepared in a registered pharmacy, hospital or health centre by or under the supervision of a pharmacist in accordance with a prescription given by a practitioner or in anticipation of such a prescription and with a view to dispensing the product.

Prepared products have a similar status to that of 'specials'. The preparing or supervising pharmacist has a professional responsibility for the inherent quality and safety of the product he supplies. These products are not, however, subjected to full quality assurance.

Unlicensed, 'Off-label', 'Off-licence'

Many drugs used for children are used outside the specification of the product licence i.e. are 'unlicensed'. The drug itself may be unlicensed, i.e. an unlicensed medicine, or it may be given by an unlicensed route of administration or for an unlicensed indication or at an unlicensed dose. There may be age limits on its use or it may be unlicensed for use in children. Sometimes the terms 'Off-label' or 'Off-licence' may be used to describe a medicine which is being used outside the specifications of the product licence.

Named patient basis

When a commercial company supplies a product for which no product licence exists, it is supplied on a named patient basis. The company will generally require a consultant's name, patient name and details of the condition which the drug will be used to treat.

Borderline substances

These are products (foods or toilet preparations) which the Advisory Committee on Borderline substances (ACBS) have stated can be regarded as drugs for the management of specified conditions, e.g. Aminogran® for phenylketonuria.

Summaries of Product Characteristics (SPCs)

SPCs are information sheets for medicinal products produced by pharmaceutical companies that follow the requirements laid down by the European Commissions' Committee for Proprietary Medicinal Products (CPMP) Note for Guidance (for SPCs).

ABBREVIATIONS

AIDS	acquired immune deficiency syndrome
AUC	area under the curve
CNS	central nervous system
CSF	cerebral spinal fluid
DNA	deoxyribonucleic acid
ECG	electrocardiogram
EEG	electroencephalogram
ETT	endotracheal tube
FBC	full blood count
G6PD	glucose 6-phosphate dehydrogenase
GFR	glomerular filtration rate
HIV	human immunodeficiency virus
IM	intramuscular
INR	international normalised ratio
IP	intraperitoneally
ITU	intensive therapy unit
IV	intravenous
JIA	juvenile idiopathic arthritis
LFT	liver function test
MAOI	monoamine-oxidase inhibitor

NaCl	sodium chloride
NSAID	non-steroidal anti-inflammatory drug
PN	parenteral nutrition
RNA	ribonucleic acid
SC	subcutaneous
SPC	summary of product characteristics
U&E	urea and electrolytes
UK	United Kingdom

Units of measurement

g	gram
hr(s)	hour (s)
kg	kilogram
kJ	kilojoules
dL	decilitre
L	litre
mg	milligram
min(s)	minute (s)
mL	millilitre
mmol	millimole
pmol	picamols
mth	month

mOsm/L	milliosmols per litre
ppm	parts per million
yr(s)	year (s)

The abbreviations yr(s), hr(s) and min(s) have only been used when absolutely necessary. Whenever possible these have not been abbreviated.

Symbols

$\geq$	greater than or equal to
$>$	greater than
$\leq$	less than or equal to
$<$	less than
$\equiv$	equivalent to
$\simeq$	approximately equal to

GLOSSARY OF SYMBOLS USED IN THE MONOGRAPHS

The following are used in the book and may be found adjacent to each drug name heading and in some cases in a smaller size within the drug's notes section.

Licensing information

 indicates that the medicine is licensed for use in all ages

 indicates that all presentations are unlicensed preparations in the UK

 indicates that the medicine is not licensed for use in children

 indicates that there are restrictions in the licensed status of the medicine. The precise nature of the restriction is explained in the notes section of the monograph.

Other symbols

 indicates either a contra-indication to use in renal impairment or that a dose adjustment is necessary due to renal impairment

 indicates either a contra-indication or a warning that the relevant preparation should be used with caution in cases of liver disease

 indicates that breast feeding is contra-indicated

The reporting of all suspected adverse drug reactions in children is strongly encouraged through the Yellow Card scheme, even if the intensive monitoring symbol (▼) has been removed, because experience in children may still be limited. Reporting is encouraged whether or not the medicine is licensed for use in children. The identification and reporting of adverse reactions to drugs in children is particularly important because:

■ The action of the drug and its disposition in children (especially in the very young), may be different from that in adults.

■ Drugs are not extensively tested in children.

■ Many drugs are not specifically licensed for use in children and are used 'off-label'.

■ Suitable formulations may not be available to allow precise dosing in children.

■ The nature and course of illnesses and adverse drug reactions may differ between adults and children.

Any drug may produce unwanted or unexpected adverse reactions. Detection and recording of these is of vital importance. Suspected adverse reactions to any therapeutic agent should be reported, including drugs (self-medication as well as prescribed ones), blood products, vaccines, x-ray contrast media, dental or surgical materials, herbal products and contact lens fluid.

Do not be put off reporting because some details are not known or if the drug has been used 'off-label' or is not licensed for use in children.

Doctors and pharmacists are urged to help by reporting adverse reactions to:

Medicines Control Agency, CSM Freepost, London SW8 5BR
Tel: 0800 731 6789

Yellow Cards for reporting can be found in *Medicines for Children*, the *British National Formulary (BNF)* and in the ABPI Compendium of Data Sheets and Summaries of Product Characteristics. For on-line reporting, please see the Medicines Control Agency* (MCA) website www.mca.gov.uk/yellowcard

A 24-hour Freephone service is available to all parts of the UK for advice and information on suspected adverse drug reactions: contact the National Yellow Card Information Service at the MCA on 0800 731 6789.

* From April 2003, the MCA merged with the Medical Devices Agency to become known as the Medicines and Healthcare Products Regulatory Agency (MHRA)

RESPIRATORY EMERGENCIES

Give oxygen to maintain saturations >95%.

Respiratory efforts present but airway obstructed - clear the airway.

Respiratory efforts absent - ventilate with bag and mask or intubate and ventilate.

Acute severe asthma

Salbutamol (100microgram/puff) up to 10 puffs via spacer and facemask or nebulise salbutamol through 7L/min oxygen (< 5 years 2.5mg, $\geq$ 5 years 5mg) and give soluble prednisolone 500 microgram/kg orally.

Acute severe croup

100% oxygen plus oral dexamethasone 150 microgram/kg.

ASYSTOLE

Before the administration of any drugs the patient must be receiving continuous and effective basic life support and ventilation with oxygen.

Ventilate with 100% oxygen, continue cardiopulmonary resuscitation- intubate and establish IV/IO access.

Adrenaline (epinephrine) 10 microgram/kg (0.1mL/kg of 1:10 000 solution) IV or IO.

Consider IV fluids and alkalising agents.

Adrenaline (epinephrine) 10-100*microgram/kg IV or IO.

Continue cardiopulmonary resuscitation, assessing every 3 minutes and repeating adrenaline if necessary.

*100 microgram/kg only where cardiac arrest is thought to have been secondary to circulatory collapse. If the patient has continuous intra-arterial monitoring the adrenaline (epinephrine) dose can be titrated to best effect. The usual second and subsequent dose will be 10 microgram/kg.

ANAPHYLAXIS

Give 100% oxygen when available.

Adrenaline (epinephrine) 1: 1000 (1mg in 1mL) IM

< 6 months	50 microgram (0.05mL)
6 months-5 years	120 microgram (0.12mL)
6-12 years	250 microgram (0.25mL)
> 12 years	500 microgram (0.5mL
	(250 microgram (0.25mL) if a small child)

Repeat after 5 minutes if no improvement.

In the presence of airway obstruction with stridor, give nebulised adrenaline (epinephrine) in addition to the IM dose.

Chlorphenamine IM or slow IV (over 1 minute)

Do not use in neonates

1 month-1 year	250 microgram/kg
1-5 years	2.5-5mg
6-12 years	5-10mg
> 12 years	10-20mg

Consider hydrocortisone IM or slow IV

< 1 year	25mg
1-5 years	50mg
6-12 years	100mg
> 12 years	200mg

FLUIDS FOR SHOCK

20mL/kg NaCl 0.9% immediately; repeat if necessary.

HYPOGLYCAEMIA

5mL/kg of 10% glucose.

ACUTE SEIZURE

Rectal diazepam

< 6 years 5mg; ≥ 6 years 10mg.

Age-mean weight and surface area for age-dose percentages

Age	Mean weight for age		Height		Body surface area	% Adult dose
	kg	lb	cm	inches	m^2	
Newborn*	3.5	7.7	50	20	0.23	12.5
1 month	4.2	9	55	22	0.26	14.5
3 months	5.6	12	59	23	0.32	18
6 months	7.7	17	67	26	0.40	22
1 year	10	22	76	30	0.47	25
3 years	15	33	94	37	0.62	33
5 years	18	40	108	42	0.73	40
7 years	23	50	120	47	0.88	50
12 years	39	86	148	58	1.25	75
Adult male	68	150	173	68	1.8	100
Adult female	56	123	163	64	1.6	100

*Full term newborn infant

The percentage adult dose method should not be used to calculate doses if paediatric doses in mg/kg or mg/m^2 are available. Newborn and preterm newborn infants may need reduced dosage.

USING WEIGHT ALONE TO CALCULATE BODY SURFACE AREA

The United Kingdom Children's Cancer Study Group (UKCCSG) Chemotherapy Standardisation group 1998 have produced tables for estimation of body surface area (based on body weight only) in infants and children. They have also produced recommendations of what percentage of calculated dose by body surface area (of cytotoxic drugs) to give to infants (≤1 year or ≤10kg). These tables and dosage recommendations can be obtained from UKCCSG or any regional paediatric cancer treatment centre.

An alternative method of calculating surface area based on body weight only is:

$$\text{Surface area (m}^2\text{)} = \frac{4 \times \text{Weight (kg)} + 7}{\text{Weight (kg)} + 90}$$

Calculation of body surface area – infants

Many nomograms underestimate the body surface area in infants and small children, therefore separate nomograms for infants (fig 1) and children (fig 2) have been included (Reprinted from *The Journal of Pediatrics*, Vol 93, Haycock et al, "Geometric method for measuring body surface area: A height-weight formula validated in infants, children and adults", pages 62-66, copyright 1978, with permission from Elsevier Science).

$$SA = W^{0.5378} \times H^{0.3964} \times 0.024265$$

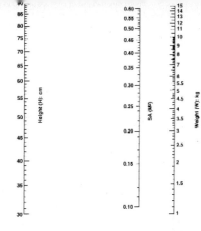

Fig 1. Nomogram representing the relationship between height, weight and body surface area in infants.

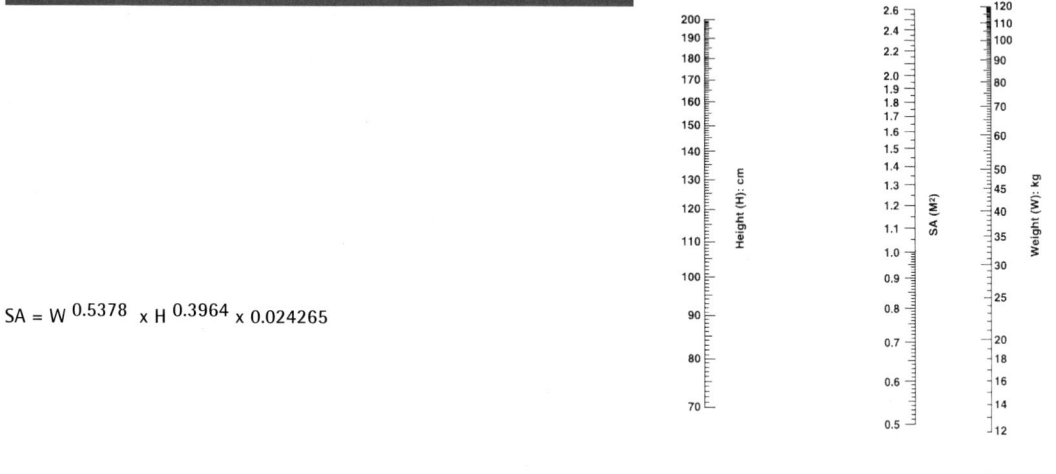

$$SA = W^{0.5378} \times H^{0.3964} \times 0.024265$$

Fig 2. Nomogram representing the relationship between height, weight and body surface area in children and adults

■ **Tablets:** 250mg.
■ **Capsules (modified release):** 250mg.

■ **Oral liquid:** may be extemporaneously prepared.
■ **Injection:** 500mg vial.

DOSAGE

Indication	Route	Age				Frequency	Notes
		birth– 1 month	1 month– 2 years	2–12 years	12–18 years	(times daily)	
Epilepsy	Oral/	←	2.5mg/kg	→	250mg	2–3	Starting dose.
	IV bolus	←	5–7mg/kg	→		2–3	Maintenance dose. Maximum dose:
					250mg	2–4	<12 years 750mg/day ≥12 years 1g/day.
Diuresis	Oral/ IV bolus	←	5mg/kg	→	250–375mg	1	
Raised intracranial pressure	Oral/ IV bolus	-	← 8mg/kg →		-	3	<u>Initial dose.</u> A gradual increase in dose may be required; doses of up to 100mg/kg/day have been used.
Glaucoma	Oral/ IV bolus	←	5mg/kg	→	250mg	2–4	Maximum dose: <12 years 750mg/day ≥12 years 1g/day.
	Oral	-	-	-	250mg	1–2	Sustained release preparation.

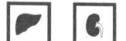

NOTES

- **Administration: oral:** injection solution is alkaline but can be diluted and given orally. **IV:** reconstitute each vial with 5mL Water for Injections and administer as a bolus.

- Chronic use may cause skin rashes and low white cell count. Monitor blood cell counts and serum electrolytes, including bicarbonate.

- Contra-indicated in liver or kidney dysfunction.

- Contra-indicated in adrenal failure, known sulphonamide hypersensitivity, low serum sodium or potassium levels and for long term use in chronic non-congestive closed angle glaucoma.

- Glaucoma and diuresis are not licensed indications in children. Raised intra-cranial pressure and epilepsy are not licensed indications.

- Increasing dose may increase incidence of paraesthesias or drowsiness without increasing diuresis.

Acetylcysteine (N-acetylcysteine, NAC)

■ **Injection**: 20% (200mg in 1mL) 10mL ampoule.

DOSAGE

Indication	Route	Age/Weight			Frequency	Notes
		under 12 years		12–18 years		
		<20 kg	>20 kg			
Treatment of paracetamol overdose	IV infusion over 15 minutes	150mg/kg in 3mL/kg	150mg/kg in 100mL	150mg/kg in 200mL	single dose	May be used up to 24 hours after paracetamol overdose. After 24 hours seek guidance from a National Poisons Information Centre.
	then	then	then	then		
	IV infusion over 4 hours	50mg/kg in 7mL/kg	50mg/kg in 250mL	50mg/kg in 500mL	single dose	
	then	then	then	then		
	IV infusion over 16 hours	100mg/kg in 14mL/kg	100mg/kg in 500mL	100mg/kg in 1 litre	single dose	

For information on use of oral acetylcysteine refer to *Medicines for Children*.

Acetylcysteine (N-acetylcysteine, NAC) continued

NOTES

■ **Administration: IV:** infuse in glucose 5%; if for any reason glucose is unsuitable, NaCl 0.9% may be substituted. A colour change to light purple is not thought to indicate significant impairment of safety or efficacy.

■ Monitoring of serum potassium is recommended as hypokalaemia may occur. Acetylcysteine may be added to potassium-containing infusion fluids.

■ High risk treatment line to be used if patient is taking liver enzyme inducing drugs (e.g. carbamazepine, phenytoin, phenobarbitol, primidone, St John's Wort or rifampicin), is a chronic alcohol abuser or has any conditions causing glutathione depletion (e.g. malnutrition, HIV infection). See graph in the paracetamol monograph in *Medicines for Children*.

■ Anaphylactoid or hypersensitivity reactions occur in up to 15% of patients. These usually resolve after stopping the infusion - occasionally antihistamines or steroids may be required.

Aciclovir (acyclovir)

■ **Tablets:** 200mg, 400mg, 800mg.
■ **Tablets (dispersible):** 200mg, 400mg, 800mg.
■ **Suspension:** 200mg in 5mL, 400mg in 5mL .

■ **Cream:** 5%.
■ **Eye ointment:** 3%.
■ **IV infusion:** 250mg, 500mg, 1g vials.

DOSAGE

Newborn infant (birth to 1 month)

Route	Age		Frequency (times daily)	Notes
	Up to 7 days	Over 7 days		
IV infusion	← 10mg/kg →		3	Usually for 10 days

Child

Herpes simplex virus treatment

Route	Age			Frequency (times daily)	Notes
	1 month–2 years	2–12 years	12–18 years		
Oral	100mg	←――― 200mg ―――→		5	Normal immune states.
	200mg	←――― 400mg ―――→		5	Severely immunocompromised or with reduced absorption.
IV infusion	<3 months 10mg/kg 3 months–2 years 250mg/m²	250mg/m²	5mg/kg	3	Normal immune states.
	<3 months 10mg/kg 3 months–2 years 500mg/m²	500mg/m²	10mg/kg	3 3	Immunocompromised or encephalitis

Herpes simplex prophylaxis

Route	Age			Frequency (times daily)	Notes
	1 month–2 years	2–12 years	12–18 years		
Oral	100mg	←――― 200mg ―――→		4	Herpes simplex prophylaxis.
	200mg	←――― 400mg ―――→		4	Severely immunocompromised.

Chickenpox and shingles treatment

Route	Age			Frequency	Notes
	1 month–2 years	2–12 years	12–18 years	(times daily)	
Oral		DOSE BY WEIGHT			Use IV route in immunocompromised for at least 5 days first.
	←	20mg/kg	→	4	
	DOSE BY AGE	DOSE BY AGE	DOSE BY AGE		
		2–5 years			
	200mg	400mg	–	4	
		6–12 years			
		800mg		4	
			800mg	5	
IV infusion	≤3 months 10mg/kg 3 months–2 years 250mg/m²	250mg/m²	5mg/kg	3	Normal immune states.
	≤3 months 10mg/kg 3 months–2 years 500mg/m²	500mg/m²	10mg/kg	3	Immunocompromised.
				3	

Dose adjustment in renal impairment

Creatinine clearance (mL/min/1.73m²)	Dose	Dose frequency
>50	normal	12 hourly
10–50	normal	daily
<10	50%	daily

Haemodialysis: dose after dialysis; dose as for creatinine clearance <10mL/min/1.73m². **CAPD**: dose as for creatinine clearance <10mL/min/1.73m².

NOTES

■ **Administration: IV:** do not give as IV bolus – if central line, reconstitute to 25mg in 1mL and give over 1 hour; if peripheral line dilute to 5mg in 1mL with NaCl 0.9% or glucose 5% and infuse over 1 hour.

■ Cream and ophthalmic ointment may be used 5 times daily. Continue eye ointment for 3 days after healing is complete.

■ Care with other nephrotoxic drugs.

■ Polyuric renal failure has occurred with high doses – ensure adequate hydration.

■ **Powder:** 25g, 50g.
■ **Granules:** 5g sachet.

■ **Suspension:** 50g pack.

DOSAGE

Route	Age			Frequency	Notes
	1 month–2 years	2–12 years	12–18 years		
Oral	← DOSE BY WEIGHT 1g/kg →			single dose	**Single dose treatment.** In most cases, charcoal should be given within one hour of ingestion.
	-	DOSE BY AGE 25–50g	50g	single dose	
	← DOSE BY WEIGHT 500mg/kg – 1g/kg →			4 hourly	**Multiple dose treatment.** Ideally continue until features of toxicity have resolved or until adverse effects of the charcoal make continued administration impracticable.
	-	DOSE BY AGE 25–50g	50g	4 hourly	

NOTES

■ If the weight/amount of poison is known, give 10 times this amount of activated charcoal - otherwise dose as in table above. If in any doubt contact a National Poisons Information Centre.

■ Because of the risk of inspiration, charcoal should never be given in the absence of a gag reflex or when there is impaired consciousness, unless the airway is first protected by an endotracheal tube.

■ Palatability of charcoal may be improved by adding blackcurrant cordial or flat cola immediately before administration.

■ Compliance may be improved by administering via a covered cup and straw.

■ **Injection:** 3mg in 1mL; 2mL vial and 10mL vial for infusion.

DOSAGE

Route	Age				Frequency	Notes
	birth–1 month	1 month–2 years	2–12 years	12–18 years		
IV bolus	← 50 microgram/kg increase after 2 minutes if necessary to 100 microgram/kg → ← → Increase further in 50 microgram/kg increments at 2 minute intervals until tachycardia terminated or to a maximum dose of: 300 microgram/kg <1 month or 500 microgram/kg >1 month.			3mg increase after 2 minutes if necessary to 6mg increase after a further 2 minutes if necessary to 12mg	single dose	Initial dose. Subsequent doses if required, as shown. Increments should not be given if high level AV block develops at any particular dose.

NOTES
■ **Administration: IV:** give into central or large peripheral vein over 2 seconds, with cardiac monitoring, followed by rapid IV flush with NaCl 0.9%.

L^R

■ **Injection:** 1 in 10,000 (100 microgram in 1mL) 10mL ampoule; 1mL, 3mL, 10mL prefilled syringe.
1 in 1,000 (1mg in 1mL) 0.5mL, 1mL ampoule; 1mL prefilled syringe.

■ **IM injection for self-administration:** 150 microgram, 300 microgram.

DOSAGE

Indication	Route	Age		Frequency	Notes
		birth–1 month			
Cardio-pulmonary resuscitation (CPR) Newborn infant	IV/ endotracheal tube (ETT)	10 microgram/kg (0.1mL/kg of 1 in 10,000)		initial dose	Endotracheal route is accepted but has unproven effectiveness in resuscitation at birth.
		10–30 microgram/kg (0.1–0.3mL/kg of 1 in 10,000)		subsequent doses	

Indication	Route	Age				Frequency	Notes
		birth–1 month	1 month–2 years	2–12 years	12–18 years		
Cardio-pulmonary resuscitation (CPR) Child	IV rapid bolus/ intraosseous	–	◄— 10 microgram/kg (0.1mL/kg of 1 in 10,000) —►		1mg (10mL of 1 in 10,000)	initial and usual subsequent dose	If given by intraosseous route, flush with 0.9% NaCl.

DOSAGE continued

Indication	Route	Age				Frequency	Notes
		birth–1 month	1 month–2 years	2–12 years	12–18 years		
Cardio-pulmonary resuscitation (CPR) Child	IV rapid bolus/intraosseous	–	←100 microgram/kg→ (0.1mL/kg of 1 in 1000 or 1mL/kg of 1 in 10,000)		5mg (5mL of 1 in 1000)	subsequent doses in exceptional circum-stances e.g. arterial monitoring, septica-emia, anaphylaxis.	Maximum dose is 5mL of 1 in 1000.
	Endotracheal tube (ETT)	–	←100 microgram/kg→ (0.1mL/kg of 1 in 1000 or 1mL/kg of 1 in 10,000)		5mg (5mL of 1 in 1000)	initial dose	If there is no venous access the ETT can be used. If there is no clinical effect, further doses should be given intravenously as soon as venous access is secured
Acute anaphylaxis	Deep IM	← 10 microgram/kg → (0.01mL/kg of 1 in 1000)			0.5–1mg (0.5–1mL of 1 in 1000)	single dose	Repeat at 5 minute intervals if necessary according to clinical response.
Low cardiac output	IV infusion	← 10 nanogram – 1 microgram/kg/minute →				continuous	Start at lower doses.
Croup	Nebulised	← 1–5mL of 1 in 1000 →			–	single dose	Produces a transient improvement, rarely alters the long term course of the illness. Observe closely with ECG and oxygen saturation monitoring.

NOTES

■ **Administration: IV:** do not use if discoloured or precipitate present. Do not mix with sodium bicarbonate. Dilute with NaCl 0.9% or glucose 5%. **ETT:** inject quickly down narrow-bore suction catheter beyond the end of the ETT and flush with 1-2mL NaCl 0.9%. **Nebulised:** dilute to 2-3mL with NaCl 0.9%.

■ Licensing varies depending on the product. See *Medicines for Children* for details.

Alfacalcidol (1α–hydroxycholecalciferol)

■ **Capsules:** 250 nanogram, 500 nanogram, 1 microgram.
■ **Oral drops:** 2 microgram in 1mL (1 drop ≈ 100 nanogram).

■ **Injection:** 2 microgram in 1mL; 0.5 mL, 1mL ampoules.

DOSAGE

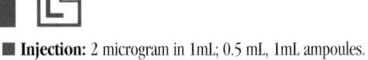

Indication	Route	Age				Frequency (times daily)	Notes
		birth– 1 month	1 month– 2 years	2–12 years	12–18 years		
Hypophos- phataemic rickets	Oral/IV	← 25–50 nanogram/kg →		<20kg 25–50 nanogram/kg >20kg 1 microgram/ dose	1 microgram/ dose	1 1	Initial dose. Adjust the dose according to response to avoid hypercalcaemia.
Neonatal hypo-	Oral/IV	50–100 nanogram/kg	–	–	–	1	Up to 2 microgram/kg may be needed in severe cases. 100 nanogram/kg/day has proven effective as prophylaxis

DOSAGE continued

Indication	Route	Age				Frequency (times daily)	Notes
		birth–1 month	1 month–2 years	2–12 years	12–18 years		
Prophylaxis of vitamin D deficiency in renal patients	Oral/IV	← 15-30 nanogram/kg →		<20kg 15–30 nanogram/kg >20kg 250–500 nanogram/dose	250–500 nanogram/dose	1 1	

NOTES

■ **Administration: oral:** measure using the dropper provided. In general the drops should not be diluted, but if necessary, may be diluted with milk immediately prior to administration; discard any remaining solution. **IV:** administer by IV bolus over 30 seconds. May be given via the return line at the end of haemodialysis.

■ Ensure adequate control of serum phosphate to reduce risk of metastatic calcification.

■ Monitor carefully for hypercalcaemia.

■ ⃞ One-Alpha® preparations are licensed for use in all ages. Alfa D® capsules are licensed for use in patients ≥20kg body weight.

■ **Tablets:** 10mg.

■ **Oral liquid:** 7.5 mg in 5mL, 30mg in 5mL.

DOSAGE

Indication	Route	Age			Frequency (times daily)	Notes
		1 month– 2 years	2–12 years	12–18 years		
Sedation	Oral	← 1.5–3mg/kg →		up to 90mg	single dose	Two hours before bedtime for night sedation or two hours prior to a procedure.
Antihistamine dose	Oral	**DOSE BY WEIGHT** <u>6 months–1 year</u> 250 microgram/kg **DOSE BY AGE** <u>≥1 year</u> 2.5mg	<u>2–4 years</u> 2.5mg <u>5-12 years</u> 5mg	– –	3–4 3–4	
		–	–	10mg	2–3	Up to a maximum of 100mg **per day**.

NOTES

■ **Administration: tablets:** the blue coating can be washed off the tablets prior to administration to enable the tablet to be more easily crushed. **Oral liquids:** may be diluted if required using simple syrup (without preservative).

■ 🄻 Licensed for use ≥2 years of age; manufacturers maximum recommended dose for premedication is 2mg/kg /dose.

■ 🄲 🄿 Avoid in patients with liver disease or severe renal impairment.

■ Avoid in patients with epilepsy or hypothyroidism.

■ **Injection:** 100mg in 2mL, 500mg in 2mL, vials.

DOSAGE

Many dose regimens exist for aminoglycosides depending on target concentrations aimed for and patient groups treated. The dose regimens below are generally accepted initial doses and dose adjustments should be made in the light of serum concentration measurement.

Divided daily dose regimen
Newborn infant (birth to 1 month)

Route	Age			Frequency	Notes
	Postconceptional age	Postnatal age	Dose	(times daily)	
IV	<35 weeks	<14 days	10mg/kg	1	Aim for a peak level (one hour post dose) of 15-30mg/L.
		>14 days	10mg/kg then 7.5mg/kg	loading dose 2	
	>35 weeks	<14 days	15mg/kg	1	
		>14 days	10mg/kg then 7.5mg/kg	loading dose 2	

Postconceptional age = gestational plus postnatal age.

Prolongation of dosage interval is recommended in neonates presenting with patent ductus arteriosus (PDA), prolonged hypoxia or treated with indometacin.

Divided daily dose regimen
Child

Route	Age			Frequency	Notes
	1 month–2 years	2–12 years	12–18 years	(times daily)	
IV or IM	←	7.5mg/kg (maximum 500mg)	→	2	Aim for a 1 hour post dose (peak) level of 15–30mg/L ≥12 years – for life threatening infection up to 1.5g/day in 3 divided doses may be given for a maximum of 10 days.
IV for cystic fibrosis patients	←	10mg/kg (maximum 500mg)	→	3	Starting dose; adjust according to drug levels. Aim for trough level of <10mg/L and 1 hour post dose (peak) level should not exceed 25–30mg/L

In patients with impaired renal function, dosage and/or frequency of administration must be adjusted in response to serum drug concentrations and the extent of renal impairment. There are various methods to determine dosage and a wide variation in dosage recommendations. See SPC for manufacturer's recommendations.

Single daily dose regimen
Newborn infant (birth–1 month)

Route	Postconceptional age/gestation*		Frequency	Notes
	32–35 weeks	>35 weeks	(times daily)	
IV	12mg/kg	15mg/kg	1	Aim for a 1 hour post dose (peak) level of 30mg/L; an 18 hour level of <3mg/L.

*Use postconceptional age if >7 days postnatal age. Postconceptional age = gestational plus postnatal age. There is little experience in neonates <32 weeks gestation. Levels

Single daily dose regimen
Child

Route	Age			Frequency	Notes
	1 month-2 years	2-12 years	12-18 years	(times daily)	
IV	←	15mg/kg	→	1	Aim for a 1 hour post dose (peak) level of 40-50mg/L; an 18 hour level of <3mg/L

Amikacin in a concentration of 2.5mg in 1mL may be used as an irrigation solution in abscess cavities, the pleural space, the peritoneum and the cerebral ventricles. See SPC for full details.

NOTES

- **Administration:** may be given IV or IM. **IV:** give as slow injection over 2-3 minutes. For larger doses and single daily dose regimens, give as an infusion over 20-30 minutes. Compatible with glucose 5% & NaCl 0.9%.

- Although amikacin is licensed for use in all ages some of the stated doses may be unlicensed; refer to SPC.

■ **Tablets:** 5mg.　　　　　　　　　　　　　　　　■ **Oral liquid:** 5mg in 5mL.

DOSAGE

Route	Age				Frequency	Notes
	birth–1 month	1 month–2 years	2–12 years	12–18 years	(times daily)	
Oral	←	200 microgram/kg	→	5–10mg	2	Prophylaxis of drug induced hypokalaemia.
	-	-	← 100 microgram/kg →		3	Nephrogenic diabetes insipidus.

NOTES

■ c Diuretic response is poor in patients with renal failure; risk of hyperkalaemia in renal impairment and when used with angiotensin-converting enzyme (ACE) inhibitors.

■ Do not use for nephrogenic diabetes insipidus in infants or young children.

■ Increased risk of nephrotoxicity with NSAIDs.

■ **Injection:** 25mg in 1mL, 10mL ampoule; 2mg in 1mL; 5mg in 1mL; 20mL ampoules. ■ Tablets (modified release): 100mg, 225mg, 350mg.

DOSAGE

Newborn infant.

Indication	Route	Age	Frequency	Notes
		birth–1 month	(times daily)	
Neonatal apnoea	IV (loading dose)	6mg/kg	1	Give over at least 20 minutes either undiluted or diluted with NaCl 0.9% or glucose 5%. Start maintenance dose 24 hours after loading dose. Monitor theophylline plasma levels. Therapeutic range 8–12mg/L. Because of the long half-life, a continuous infusion is not necessary.
	IV (maintenance dose)	2.5mg/kg	2	

Child

Indication	Route	Age			Frequency	Notes
		1 month–2 years	2–12 years	12–18 years		
Diuresis in intensive care	IV infusion over 20–30 minutes	← 2–4mg/kg →		–	single dose	Synergistic effect if given 30 minutes before IV furosemide (frusemide). Doses of up to 6mg/kg have been used in critically ill children.

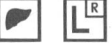

Child continued

Indication	Route	Age			Frequency	Notes
		1 month–2 years	2–12 years	12–18 years	(times daily)	
Bronchodilator in asthma or anaphylaxis	IV infusion over 20–30 minutes	⟵	5mg/kg (maximum 500mg)	⟶	single loading dose over 20–30 minutes	Loading dose if no theophylline or aminophyline has been given in the last 24 hours.
	IV infusion	⟵	1mg/kg/hour ⟶	500 microgram/kg/hour	continuous	Maintenance dose. Infusion can usually be stopped and not tapered down.
	Oral	–	≥3 years 6mg/kg* for 1 week then 12mg/kg	100–225mg for 1 week then 200–450mg	2 2	*Round doses to nearest 100mg dose. Some children with chronic asthma may need 13–20mg/kg twice daily.

NOTES

■ **Administration: IV infusion:** dilute infusion to 1mg in 1mL in NaCl 0.9% (preferred diluent), or glucose 5%. The infusion can usually be stopped and not tapered down. Give via a rate controlled infusion device. If patient is fluid-restricted, injection solution can be given undiluted. **Oral:** swallow tablets whole, do not chew.

■ 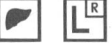 Clearance of aminophylline can decrease (and therefore blood levels increase) with reduced hepatic or cardiac function. Maintenance dose should be halved.

■ Therapeutic range in asthma therapy is 10-20mg/L (55-110 micromol/L).

■ Has a narrow therapeutic range – significant side-effects can occur when level is >14mg/L in a neonate and >20mg/L in older children

■ Breast-feeding is not contra-indicated but it is recommended that a mother feeds her baby just prior to taking her next dose, when plasma theophylline levels are expected to be low.

■ Neonatal apnoea and diuresis are unlicensed indications. The 2mg in 1mL and 5mg in 1mL injections are available as 'specials' and are therefore unlicensed.

Amiodarone hydrochloride

■ **Tablets:** 100mg, 200mg.
■ **Oral liquid:** manufactured 'special' or may be extemporaneously prepared.

■ **Injection:** 30mg in 1mL, 10mL prefilled syringe; 50mg in 1mL; 3mL ampoule.

DOSAGE

Route	Age				Frequency (times daily)	Notes
	birth–1 month	1 month–2 years	2–12 years	12–18 years		
Oral (loading dose)	←	5mg/kg (maximum 200mg)	→		2–3	Give loading dose for 7-14 days (some neonatologists use a loading dose of 10mg/kg once daily), then reduce to minimum effective maintenance dose.
				200mg	3	
Oral (maintenance dose)	←	5mg/kg (maximum 200mg)	→		1	
				200mg	1	

Child continued

Route	Frequency	Age				Notes
	(times daily)	birth–1 month	1 month–2 years	2–12 years	12–18 years	
IV (loading dose)	single dose	5mg/kg ← →				Slow IV injection over 30 minutes. Loading doses up to 15mg/kg have been reported. Give via a central line where possible. Adjust rate according to clinical response.
IV infusion	continuous	5–15 microgram/kg/minute ← → (maximum 1.2g in 24 hours)				In cardiopulmonary resuscitation (CPR) for shock resistant ventricular fibrillation and pulseless tachycardia.
Rapid IV bolus	single dose	5mg/kg ← → (maximum 300mg)				

NOTES

■ **Administration: oral:** tablets are scored. It is possible to crush tablets and disperse in water. However an oral suspension may be extemporaneously prepared. **IV:** amiodarone may be administered more rapidly in emergency situations as a slow IV injection over at least 3 minutes at a concentration of 15mg in 1mL in glucose 5%. This should not be repeated for at least 15 minutes. Injection is compatible with glucose 5% only. Solutions containing less than 150mg of amiodarone in 250mL glucose 5% (600 microgram in 1mL) are unstable and should not be used.

■ Use is contra-indicated where there is evidence or history of thyroid dysfunction, sinus bradycardia and sino-atrial heart block. IV amiodarone use is contra-indicated in severe respiratory failure, circulatory collapse or severe arterial hypotension.

■ Dosage adjustment should be considered in liver disease.

■ Maintenance doses of digoxin should be halved when given in combination with amiodarone.

■ Dosage adjustment (of amiodarone or the interacting drug) should be considered when amiodarone is used in combination with: beta-blockers, calcium channel blockers, phenytoin, cimetidine, ciclosporin, oral anticoagulant therapy, antiarrhythmics, agents which may induce hypokalaemia and/or hypomagnesaemia, and general anaesthesia. See *Medicines for Children* for details.

■ Use with caution when administering to patients with a known hypersensitivity to iodine.

■ Use with caution in patients with heart failure.

Amitriptyline

■ **Tablets:** 10mg, 25mg, 50mg.
■ **Capsules:** 25mg, 50 mg.
■ **Oral solution:** 10mg in 5mL, 25mg in 5mL, 50mg in 5mL.

DOSAGE

Indication	Route	Age		Frequency	Notes
		2–12 years	12–18 years	(times daily)	
Nocturnal enuresis	Oral	≥ 6 years 10–25mg	25–50mg	1 (at night)	Unlikely to be indicated <6 years. Maximum period of treatment 3 months – review before further courses.
Depression	Oral	–	25mg or 50mg	2–3 1 (at night)	Initial dose. Start at the lower dose and increase as tolerated if required. Usual maintenance dose 50–100mg daily.

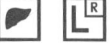

DOSAGE continued

Indication	Route	Age		Frequency	Notes
		2–12 years	12–18 years	(times daily)	
Neuralgic pain	Oral	–	30mg	1 (at night)	<u>Initial dose.</u> Start at this dose and increase as tolerated if required up to 150mg daily.
Idiopathic musculoskeletal pain	Oral	> 8 years 10–50mg	10–50mg	1 (at night)	Start at the lower dose and increase as tolerated if required.

NOTES

- Tricyclic antidepressants lower the seizure threshold and should be used with caution in patients with a history of convulsions. They may also increase the risk of arrhythmias and should be avoided in patients with heart block or a history of arrhythmias.

- Increased risk of ventricular arrhythmias with amiodarone and terfenadine; avoid concomitant use.

- Treatment should be withdrawn gradually.

- Use with caution in liver disease; avoid if severe.

- Licensed for treatment of depression ≥16 years of age and enuresis ≥6 years of age. Neuralgic pain is not a licensed indication.

■ **Capsules:** 250mg, 500mg.
■ **Syrup:** 125mg in 5mL, 250mg in 5mL.
■ **Suspension:** 125mg in 5mL, 250mg in 5mL.

■ **Paediatric suspension:** 125mg in 1.25mL.
■ **Sachets:** 3g.
■ **Injection:** 250mg, 500mg, 1g vials.

DOSAGE

Newborn infant (birth to 1 month)

Route	Age	Dose	Frequency	Notes
Oral/IV/IM	<7 days	50mg/kg	12 hourly	Increase IV dose to 100mg/kg in suspected meningitis.
	7–21 days	50mg/kg	8 hourly	
	>21 days	50mg/kg	6 hourly	

Child

Route	Age			Frequency (times daily)	Notes
	1 month–2 years	2–12 years	12–18 years		
Oral	DOSE BY WEIGHT ← 8mg/kg →		-	3	Dose may be doubled in severe infection.
	DOSE BY AGE 125mg	125–250mg	500mg	3	
IV/IM	← 30mg/kg →			3	Dose may be doubled in severe infection/meningitis up to a maximum **daily** dose of 4g.

Child continued

Route	Age			Frequency (times daily)	Notes
	1 month–2 years	2–12 years	12–18 years		
Oral for cystic fibrosis patients	⟵	**DOSE BY WEIGHT** 16–33mg/kg	⟶	3	Treatment for asymptomatic *Haemophilus influenzae* carriage or mild exacerbations.
		DOSE BY AGE			
	≤1 year 125mg	≤7 years 250mg	500mg	3	
	≥1 year 250mg	≥7 years 500mg		3	
Oral for *H. pylori*	>1 year 125mg	2–6 years 125mg	500mg		Treatment for 14 days with metronidazole and omeprazole.
		6–12 years 250mg		3	
	>1 year 250mg	2–6 years 250mg	1g	2	Treatment for 14 days with clarithromycin and omeprazole.
		6–12 years 500mg		2	

Dose adjustment in renal impairment

Creatinine clearance (mL/min/1.73m²)	Dose	Dose frequency
>50	normal	normal
10-50	normal	12 hourly
<10	normal	18 hourly

Amoxicillin is removed by haemodialysis and peritoneal dialysis. In dialysis patients a dose should be given after dialysis session; give dose as per creatinine clearance of 10-50mL/min/1.73m² in above table.

NOTES

■ **Administration: IV:** reconstitute with Water for Injections - 250mg vial with 4.8mL to give 50mg in 1mL; 500mg vial with 9.6mL to give 50mg in 1mL; 1g vial with 19.2mL to give 50mg in 1mL. Some neonatal units reconstitute 250mg with 2.4mL and 500mg with 4.8mL each giving 100mg in 1mL. Give over 3-5 minutes; higher doses over 30 minutes.

■ Compatible with glucose 5% and 10%, and with NaCl 0.45% and 0.9%.

■ **IV infusion lipid formulations:** amphotericin B lipid complex 5mg in 1mL, 10 & 20mL vials – Abelcet®; amphotericin B cholesteryl sulphate complex 50mg, 100mg vials – Amphocil®.

■ **Liposomal amphotericin:** 50mg vial – AmBisome®.
■ **IV infusion:** 50mg vial – Fungizone®.

DOSAGE
Newborn infant

Preparation	Route	Age	Frequency	Notes
		birth to 1 month	(times daily)	
Conventional formulation	IV	250 microgram/kg	1	See test dose recommendations in notes section p31. Increase by 250 microgram/kg once daily (up to a maximum 1mg/kg/day in severe infections).
Liposomal formulation	IV	1mg/kg increasing by 1mg/kg/day to 3mg/kg or 5mg/kg	1 1 1	See test dose recommendations in notes section, p31. Empirical treatment. Proven systemic infection.

Child

Preparation	Route	Age			Frequency (times daily)	Notes
		1 month-2 years	2-12 years	12-18 years		
Conventional formulation	IV	←	250 microgram/kg increase by 250 microgram/kg/day to	→	1	See test dose recommendations. in notes section p31. Adjust according to response and tolerance.
		←	1mg/kg	→	1	If therapy interrupted for longer than 7 days, restart at low dose and increase as previously. Maximum dose is 1.5mg/kg/day.
Liposomal formulation	IV	←	1mg/kg increase by 1mg/kg/day to	→	1	See test dose recommendations in notes section p31.
		←	3mg/kg or	→	1	Empirical.
		←	5mg/kg	→	1	Proven systemic infection.

Child continued

Preparation	Route	Age			Frequency	Notes
		1 month-2 years	2-12 years	12-18 years	(times daily)	
Liposomal formulation	IV	←	1-3mg/kg/day for 10-21 days to a cumulative dose of 21-30mg/kg	→	1	Visceral leishmaniasis in immunocompetent patients.
		←	3mg/kg	→	1 on days 1–5, and days 14 and 21	Visceral leishmaniasis in immunocompetent patients. (USA guidance).
Lipid formulations	IV	←	1mg/kg increase by 1mg/kg/day to	→	1	See test dose recommendations in notes section p31.
		←	3mg/kg or	→	1	Empirical.
		←	5mg/kg	→	1	Proven systemic infection.

Child continued

Preparation	Route	Age			Frequency (times daily)	Notes
		1 month–2 years	2–12 years	12–18 years		
Conventional formulation	Nebulised	–	≤10 years 5mg ≥10 years 10mg	10mg	2 2	
	Bladder irrigation	← 50–100 microgram in 1mL solution →			2	Use appropriate volume.

NOTES

■ **Administration:** consult *Medicines for Children* or product literature for full details of reconstitution, dilution, compatibility with infusion fluids etc before administration.

■ Monitor serum potassium, magnesium and phosphate carefully as low serum levels may occur.

■ Administer a test dose before each new treatment course – 100 microgram/kg (maximum 1mg) over 30 minutes for the conventional formulation or 10-15 minutes for the other formulations; observe for anaphylaxis over 30 minutes, then continue treatment.

■ ⃞ⁱᴱ All formulations unlicensed for use in neonates. Maximum licensed daily dosage of liposomal amphotericin is 3mg/kg. IV infusion preparations are not licensed for nebulisation.

■ ⃞ᶜ No dose reduction is generally required in pre-existing renal impairment. Dose reduction may be advisable if amphotericin is suspected of causing nephrotoxicity. Lipid complex formulations should also be considered in such situations. In renal dialysis patients, administration of amphotericin should commence only when dialysis is completed.

32 Ampicillin

- **Capsules:** 250mg, 500mg.
- **Syrup:** 125mg in 5mL, 250mg in 5mL.
- **Injection:** 500mg vial.

DOSAGE

Newborn infant (birth to 1 month)

Route	Age	Dose	Frequency	Notes
Oral/IV/IM	<7 days	50mg/kg	12 hourly	Increase IV dose to 100mg/kg/dose in suspected meningitis or Group B streptococcal infection.
	7-21 days	50mg/kg	8 hourly	
	>21 days	50mg/kg	6 hourly	

Child

Route	Age			Frequency (times daily)	Notes
	1 month-2 years	2-12 years	12-18 years		
Oral	12.5mg/kg	250mg	500mg	4	
IV/IM	← 25mg/kg →			4	Maximum single dose 1g.
IV infusion	← 100mg/kg →			4	Septicaemia, CNS or severe infection. Maximum single dose 3g.

Dose adjustment in renal impairment

Creatinine clearance (mL/min/1.73m²)	Dose	Dose frequency
>50	normal	8 hourly
10-50	normal	8-12 hourly
<10	normal	daily

Ampicillin is removed by haemodialysis and peritoneal dialysis. Patients undergoing dialysis should receive a dose of ampicillin after dialysis session.
CAPD: dose as for creatinine clearance of 10-50mL/min/1.73m² in the above table.

NOTES

■ **Administration: IV:** for IV administration, reconstitute the 500mg vial with 9.6mL Water for Injections to give 50mg in 1mL. Some units reconstitute with 4.6mL to get a solution containing 100mg in 1mL. Administer as a slow IV injection over 3-5 minutes or inject into flowing infusion. High dose therapy (100mg/kg) may need to be infused over at least 10 minutes due to the volume administered. Compatible with glucose 5% & 10% & glucose/saline combinations but must be used within 1 hour. Incompatible with dextrans, lipid emulsions, sodium bicarbonate. Do not mix with aminoglycosides: adequate flushing between doses or administration at separate sites is recommended.

■ **Tablets (dispersible, enteric coated):** 75 mg, 300mg.

DOSAGE

Indication	Route	Age			Frequency	Notes
		1 month–2 years	2–12 years	12–18 years	(times daily)	
Anti-platelet dose	Oral	←——— 10mg/kg ———→		75mg	1	
Kawasaki disease	Oral	←——— 25mg/kg ———→ then		–	4	Give the higher dose until the 14th day of illness or until afebrile, followed by a single daily dose of 5mg/kg for 6-8 weeks for all patients. If no evidence of coronary lesions, discontinue after this period, otherwise seek cardiology opinion.
		←——— 5mg/kg ———→		–	1	

NOTES

■ **Administration:** to give doses less than 75 mg, dissolve one tablet in 10-15 mL of water and use a proportion to obtain correct dose. Use immediately and discard remainder.

■ Contra-indicated in active peptic ulceration, haemophilia & other bleeding disorders. Should not be given to children <16 years as analgesic/antipyretic (risk of Reye's syndrome).

■ Increased risk of bleeding with anticoagulants, decreased excretion of methotrexate, enhanced effect of phenytoin and sodium valproate.

■ **Tablets:** 25mg, 50mg, 100mg.   ■ **Syrup:** 25mg in 5mL.

DOSAGE

Route	Age				Frequency (times daily)	Notes
	birth–1 month	1 month–2 years	2–12 years	12–18 years		
Oral	←	1–2mg/kg	→	50mg	1	Adjust according to blood pressure and heart rate. May be given twice daily if necessary.

NOTES

■ Avoid in patients with a history of asthma and in heart failure.

■ No dose adjustment is required in patients with a creatinine clearance >35mL/min/1.73m^2. If creatinine clearance 10-35mL/min/1.73m^2 give 50% dose, <10mL/min/1.73m^2 give 30-50% dose and adjust according to

response. In haemodialysis and CAPD give 30-50% of dose and adjust according to response.

■ See propranolol monograph in *Medicines for Children* for further information about side-effects and interactions.

■ **Injection:** 10mg in 1mL; 2.5mL, 5mL and 25mL ampoules.

DOSAGE

Route	Age				Frequency	Notes
	birth–1 month	1 month–2 years	2–12 years	12–18 years		
IV bolus	300–500 microgram/kg	←	300–600 microgram/kg	→	single dose	Initial dose. Supplemental doses of 100–200 microgram/kg can be given. (Up to 1mg/kg for rapid sequence induction).
IV infusion	300–400 microgram/kg/hour	300–600 microgram/kg/hour (5–10 microgram/kg/minute)			continuous	

NOTES

■ **Administration: IV:** IV infusion should be at a concentration of ≥500 microgram in 1mL in glucose 5% or NaCl 0.9% (both stable for 24 hours).

■ Non-cumulative effect and only effective for 15–30 minutes.

■ There is little published information on use in newborn infants who may be more sensitive to atracurium than children and adults.

■ 🔲 Licensed for use ≥1 month of age.

■ **Injection:** 600 microgram in 1mL; 1mL ampoule (other strengths available). 100 microgram in 1mL; 5mL, 10mL and 30mL disposable syringes. 200 microgram in 1mL; 5mL disposable syringe.

300 microgram in 1mL; 10mL disposable syringe.
■ **Oral solution:** 500 microgram in 5mL – available as a 'special'.

DOSAGE

Route	Age				Frequency	Notes
	birth–1 month	1 month–2 years	2–12 years	12–18 years		
SC/IM	15 microgram/kg	← 10–30 microgram/kg → (minimum 100 microgram, maximum 600 microgram)		300–600 microgram	single dose	Not to be given IM in neonates. Administer 45 minutes before procedure.
IV bolus over 1 minute	15 microgram/kg	← 20 microgram/kg → (minimum 100 microgram, maximum 600 microgram)		300–600 microgram	single dose	Dose to be given at induction in the unpremedicated.
Oral	← 20–40 microgram/kg → (maximum 900 microgram)			900 microgram	single dose	Administer 1–2 hours pre-operatively.

NOTES

■ Contra-indications: urinary tract obstruction, ileus, pyloric stenosis, glaucoma.

■ 🅛 The oral solution is available as a 'special' from Rosemont, and is therefore unlicensed.

- **Tablets:** 25mg, 50mg.
- **Oral liquid:** may be extemporaneously prepared.
- **Injection:** 50mg vial.
- **Capsule:** 10mg - manufactured 'special'.

DOSAGE

Route	Age			Frequency (times daily)	Notes
	1 month–2 years	2–12 years	12–18 years		
Oral/IV	←	1.5–3mg/kg	→	1	The total daily oral dose may be given in 2 divided doses. Only use IV when the oral route is impractical.
Oral	←	2mg/kg	→	1	Inflammatory bowel disease. The total daily dose may be given in 2 divided doses.

NOTES

- During the first 4 weeks of therapy, full blood count (including platelets) should be performed at least weekly, and monthly thereafter.
- **R** Dose should be reduced in renal failure.
- In transplantation, dose depends on the immunosuppressive regimen employed: always follow the protocol.
- If allopurinol and azathioprine are used together then the azathioprine dose should be reduced to one quarter of the usual dose.
- **L R** Licensed for use in children and adults, but not for inflammatory bowel disease. Capsule is a 'special' and as such is unlicensed.
- Capsule available from Nova Laboratories.

■ **Capsules:** 250mg.
■ **Tablets:** 500mg.

■ **Suspension:** 200mg in 5mL; 15mL, 22.5mL, 30mL.

DOSAGE

Route	Age			Frequency (times daily)	Notes
	1 month–2 years	2–12 years	12–18 years		
Oral	◄——— DOSE BY WEIGHT ———►				For 3 days.
	>6 months 10mg/kg	10mg/kg	–	1	Continued treatment may be necessary to prevent relapse in cryptosporidiosis.
		◄——— DOSE BY AGE ———►			
		3–7 years 200mg	12–14 years 400mg	1	
		8–11 years 300mg	>14 years 500mg	1	
	–	–	1g	single dose	Sexually transmitted diseases caused by *Chlamydia trachomatis*.
Oral for cystic fibrosis patients	◄——— 10mg/kg ———► (maximum dose 500mg)		500mg	1 for 3 days	Treatment of asymptomatic *S. aureus* isolates or minor exacerbations; asymtomatic *H. influenzae* carriage or mild exacerbation; atypical infection e.g. Mycoplasma. Repeat course one week later and then repeat as necessary.

NOTES

 Avoid in liver disease.

■ 🅛 Licensed for use in adults and children >6 months of age.

■ **Tablets:** 10mg.

■ **Oral liquid:** 5mg in 5ml.

■ **Intrathecal injection:** 50 microgram in 1ml, 1ml ampoule; 500 microgram in 1ml, 20ml ampoule; 2mg in 1ml, 5ml ampoule - Lioresal®; 1mg in 1ml, 2ml, 12 ml vials; 3 mg in 1ml, 12ml vial ('specials').

DOSAGE

Route	Age			Frequency (times daily)	Notes
	1 month–2 years	2–12 years	12–18 years		
Oral					
	≥1 year 2.5mg	2.5mg	5mg	3	Initial dose. Increase gradually every 3 days to maintenance doses.
	-	10–20mg	3		Maintenance dose. Maximum **daily dose** 100mg.
	≥1 year 5–10mg	2–6 years 6–10 years 10–15mg 15–30mg >10 years as 12–18 years	2		Maintenance dose. Doses are shown for a twice daily regimen; the total daily dose can be given as 2, 3 or 4 divided doses.
Intrathecal	-	≥4 years 25–50 microgram	25–50 microgram	single dose	Test dose. Maintenance doses are titrated according to individual need.

NOTES

■ **Administration: oral:** the liquid may be diluted with Purified Water BP and stored at room temperature for up to 14 days. If nausea is a problem, despite dose reduction, then baclofen may be ingested with food or milk. **Intrathecal:** the 50 microgram in 1mL intrathecal injection is intended for administration as a test via a lumbar puncture or intrathecal catheter. The other preparations are intended to be given by implantable pumps in experienced centres - see manufacturer's SPC for details.

■ **C** Reduce oral dose by at least 50% in patients with impaired renal function and the frequency to 3 times daily (mild), twice daily (moderate) or daily (severe).

■ Drug withdrawal should be gradual over at least 1-2 weeks.

■ Use with caution in epilepsy.

■ **L** Licensed for oral use ≥1 year of age. Lioresal® injection is licensed in adults and children for treatment of spasticity of cerebral origin only. It is not licensed <18 years of age for treatment of spasticity of spinal origin. The 1mg in 1mL and the 3mg in 1mL injections are 'specials' and therefore unlicensed.

■ The 1mg in 1mL and 3mg in 1mL intrathecal injections are available as 'specials' from Victoria Pharmaceuticals, The Royal Hospitals, Belfast.

Beclometasone (beclomethasone) dipropionate

■ **Aerosol inhaler:** 50, 100, 200, 250 microgram per actuation.
■ **CFC-free inhaler (metered dose and Autohaler®):** 50, 100 microgram per actuation – Qvar®.
■ **Breath-actuated inhaler:** 50, 100, 250 microgram per actuation.

■ **Dry powder devices:** 100, 200, 400 microgram per blister/capsule – Becodisks®
■ **Dry powder inhaler:** 50, 100, 250 microgram per actuation.
■ **Nasal spray:** 50 microgram per metered spray.

DOSAGE

Route	Age			Frequency (times daily)	Notes
	1 month–2 years	2–12 years	12–18 years		
Aerosol inhaler	>6 months 50–200 microgram	← 100–400 microgram →		2	Asthma: preventor for regular use **a smaller dose of Qvar® may be required.
Dry powder inhalation	–	← >5 years 100–400 microgram →		2	Asthma: preventor – for regular use.
Intra-nasal	–	← >6 years 100 microgram (2 sprays) → into each nostril		2	Allergic rhinitis.

** A dose reduction may be needed when switching patients to Qvar® from a CFC-containing beclometasone preparation. This is because Qvar® is formulated as an 'extra-fine' aerosol which is said to deposit more drug in the lungs than conventional formulations. Patients with well controlled asthma may require a smaller dose of Qvar® as compared with conventional formulations. Poorly controlled patients may be switched at the same microgram for microgram dose, up to 800 microgram daily.

NOTES

■ Metered dose inhalers are compatible with the Volumatic® spacer device. The CFC-free presentation is compatible with the Aerochamber® spacer device.

■ Rinse mouth well after use to reduce hoarseness and throat irritation. Wash face after use of mask.

■ When switching from CFC-containing to CFC-free aerosols, a lower dose may continue to offer control.

■ [L] All products are licensed for use in children with the exception of inhalers of strength >200 microgram per actuation and the CFC-free presentations; the maximum licensed dose in children is 400 microgram per day.

Bendroflumethiazide (bendrofluazide)

■ **Tablets:** 2.5mg, 5mg.

■ **Oral liquid:** may be extemporaneously prepared.

DOSAGE

Route	Age			Frequency (times daily)	Notes
	1 month–2 years	2–12 years	12–18 years		
Oral	← 50–100 microgram/kg →		2.5–5mg	1	Maintenance dose. In children doses up to 400 microgram/kg may be needed initially, reducing to the maintenance dose.

Bendroflumethiazide (bendrofluazide) continued

NOTES

■ When creatinine clearance falls below 30ml/min/1.73m², thiazide diuretics become ineffective. Contra-indicated in severe renal failure.

■ See chlorothiazide monograph for further information.

■ Tablets are licensed for use in children and adults but the liquid needs to be extemporaneously prepared and is therefore unlicensed.

Benzylpenicillin (penicillin G)

■ **Injection:** 600mg and 1.2g vials.

DOSAGE

Newborn infant (birth to 1 month)

Route	Age		Frequency (times daily)	Notes
	Up to 7 days	Over 7 days		
IV	25mg/kg	-	2	Doses should be doubled when there is evidence of
IV	-	25mg/kg	3	meningitis (especially group B streptococcal meningitis).

Child

Route	Age			Frequency (times daily)	Notes
	1 month–2 years	2–12 years	12–18 years		
IV	←	25mg/kg	→	4	
	←	50mg/kg	→	6	In severe infection (including meningitis) doses of 50mg/kg may be given 6 times daily; maximum single dose 2.4g, maximum 14.4g/**day**.

Dose adjustment in renal impairment

Creatinine clearance (mL/min/1.73m²)	Dose	Dose frequency
>50	normal	normal
10–50	normal	8–12 hourly
<10	normal	12 hourly

Benzylpenicillin is moderately dialysed. Dose after haemodialysis. CAPD: dose as for creatinine clearance <10mL/min/1.73m² in the above table.

NOTES

■ **Administration:** on reconstitution 600mg of powder displaces 0.4mL. **IV:** for IV injection, dissolve 600mg in 4-10mL Water for Injections. For IV infusion, dissolve 600mg in at least 10mL NaCl 0.9% or Water for Injections and give over 10-30 minutes. Give doses of 50mg/kg by infusion to avoid CNS toxicity and convulsions.

■ **Tablets (enteric-coated):** 5mg.

■ **Suppositories:** 5mg, 10mg.

DOSAGE

Indication	Route	Age			Frequency (times daily)	Notes
		1 month–2 years	2–12 years	12–18 years		
Constipation	Oral	5mg	<10 years 5mg >10 years 5-10mg	5-10mg	1 1	Give tablets at night. May be necessary to increase up to 15-20mg once daily.
	Rectal	5mg	<10 years 5mg >10 year 10mg	10mg	1 1	Give suppositories in the morning.
Preparation for radiological examination	Oral (and rectal if necessary – see notes)	5mg	<10 years 5mg >10 years 10mg	10mg	1 1	Oral dose on each of the 2 nights before the investigation and rectal dose, if necessary, 1 hour before investigation.

NOTES

■ Enteric-coated tablets are designed to disintegrate in the intestine and must be swallowed without crushing or chewing.

■ Tablets taken after food act in 10-12 hours; suppositories produce a response within 60 minutes.

SPECIAL NOTE BOWEL CLEANSING SOLUTIONS ARE NOT LICENSED AS TREATMENTS FOR CONSTIPATION.

Picolax® – sodium picosulfate (sodium picosulphate)

■ **Oral powder:** 16.5g of powder per sachet (sodium picosulfate 10mg).

DOSAGE

Route	Age			Notes
	1 month–2 years	2–12 years	12–18 years	
Oral	≥1 year ¼ sachet am and ¼ sachet pm	2–4 years ½ sachet am and ½ sachet pm 4–9 years 1 sachet am and ½ sachet pm ≥9 years as for 12–18 years	1 sachet am and 1 sachet pm	Take on day prior to examination; first dose before 8am and second dose between 2pm and 4pm.

NOTES

■ **Administration: oral:** dissolve contents of sachet in 25mL water – the solution will become hot. After 5 minutes, dilute to 150mL and swallow the required amount.

■ Onset of effect is about 3 hours after the first dose.

■ 🅛 Licensed for use in adults and children ≥ 1year of age.

Klean-prep®

■ **Oral powder:** polyethylene glycol 59g, anhydrous sodium phosphate 5.685g, sodium bicarbonate 1.685g, sodium chloride 1.465g, potassium chloride 0.7425g per sachet.

DOSAGE

Orally or via nasogastric tube: 10mL/kg/hour for 30 minutes then 20mL/kg/hour for 30 minutes then increase to 25mL/kg/hour if well tolerated. Maximum volume is 100mL/kg (or 4 litres whichever is smaller) over 4 hours. Patients must be reviewed at 4 hours when, if the output is not yet clean, a further 4 hours treatment may be prescribed. Maximum total volume over 8 hours is 200mL/kg (or 8 litres whichever is the smaller amount) unless further treatment is approved by the consultant or deputy.

NOTES
■ Add contents of each sachet to 1 litre of water.

■ Older children may drink the required quantity every 10-15 minutes.

■ May be administered via a nasogastric tube.

■ Monitor for fluid overload or dehydration and electrolyte disturbance.

■ 🔲 Not licensed for use in children of less than 20kg in weight.

Citramag®

■ **Oral powder:** each sachet contains an effervescent powder which produces 17.7g magnesium citrate in aqueous solution.

DOSAGE

Oral: 5–9 years: one third of a sachet, **10–12 years:** half a sachet, **12–18 years:** one sachet; before the examination or surgery.

NOTES
■ Hot water is needed to prepare the solution. Cool before drinking. See
patient information leaflet or SPC for details of magnesium salt
administration.

■ 🔲 Licensed for use in adults and children ≥5 years of age.

■ **Aerosol inhaler:** 50, 200 microgram per actuation.
■ **Dry powder inhaler:** 100, 200, 400 microgram per actuation.
■ **Nebuliser solution:** 500 microgram in 2mL, 1mg in 2mL.

■ **Capsules:** 3mg .
■ **Capsules (modified release):** 3mg .
■ **Enema:** 2mg in 100mL .

DOSAGE
Birth to 4 months

Indication	Route	Age	Frequency	Notes
		Birth–4 months	(times daily)	
Prophylaxis and management of BPD	Inhaled (spacer)	400 microgram/kg	2	For ventilated babies.
	Inhaled (nebuliser)	500 microgram	2	For non-ventilated babies. May be increased to 1mg twice daily in babies >2.5kg with severe symptoms.

Child

Indication	Route	Age			Frequency (times daily)	Notes
		1 month–2 years	2–12 years	12–18 years		
Prophylaxis of asthma	Aerosol	← 50–400 microgram →		200–400 microgram	2	Preventor, for regular use. Can use up to 800 micrograms/day in periods of severe asthma.
	Turbohaler	-	← 100–400 microgram →		2	
	Nebuliser	← ≥ 3 months 250–500 microgram →		500 microgram – 1mg	2	Higher doses have been used.
Croup	Nebuliser	← 2mg →			single dose	
Crohn's disease	Oral m/r capsules	Not recommended		9mg	once in the morning	For up to 8 weeks, reducing the dose in the last 2–4 weeks. Induction of remission in mild to moderate disease affecting the ileum and/or the ascending colon.
	Oral	Not recommended		3mg	3	
Ulcerative colitis	Rectal	Not recommended		1 enema	once nightly	For 4 weeks. Rectal and recto-sigmoid disease.

NOTES

■ **Administration: Inhaler:** aerosol inhaler can be used via Nebuhaler® and mask for infants and young children. **Inhalation via spacer:** in ventilated babies use a spacer of approximately 145mL (Aerochamber®) attached directly to the ET tube. Hand ventilate the baby using a bag system via the Aerochamber®. Once chest movement is established activate the metered dose device and then inflate the chest ten times for each dose.

■ Rinse mouth well after use to reduce hoarseness and throat irritation. Wash face after use of mask.

■ Respules® can be diluted with NaCl 0.9% or mixed with terbutaline or ipratropium nebuliser solutions.

■ Capsules should be swallowed whole or opened and granules taken in apple/orange juice without chewing.

■ Nebulised therapy for asthma licensed ≥3 months of age. Enema and capsules are not licensed for use in children.

Bupivacaine hydrochloride

L

■ **Injection:** 0.25%, 0.375%, 0.5%, 0.75% in 10mL ampoule.

DOSAGE

Route	Age				Frequency	Notes
	birth-1 month	1 month-2 years	2-12 years	12-18 years	(times daily)	
Local infiltration	←	up to 0.8mL/kg of 0.25% (up to 2mg/kg)	→	up to 60mL of 0.25% (up to 150mg)	single dose	Do not administer more than every 8 hours.

For details on epidural administration see *Medicines for Children*. Epidural administration should be carried out by, or under the supervision of, a consultant anaesthetist.

NOTES

■ Contra-indicated in IV regional anaesthesia (Biers block), complete heart block and hypovolaemia.

■ **Oral liquid:** 10mg in 1mL, 20mg in 1mL.

■ **Injection:** 5mg in 1mL, 2mL ampoule; 10mg in 1mL, 1mL, 2mL, 5mL ampoules. 25mg in 1mL, 2mL ampoule; 50mg in 1mL, 10mL ampoule.

DOSAGE

Route	Age	Frequency (times daily)	Notes
	birth–3 months		
IV or oral loading dose	20mg/kg	single dose	
IV or oral maintenance dose	5mg/kg	1	Start maintenance dose 24 hours after loading dose. Some babies need 10mg/kg this dose twice daily if more than 44 weeks postconceptional age.

NOTES

■ Usual therapeutic range is 10–20mg/L (caffeine base) but levels of 25–35mg/L are occasionally needed. Monitoring is not necessary at standard dosage.

■ UL All the preparations are unlicensed and available as 'specials' from various 'specials' manufacturers.

■ **THE DOSES IN THE TABLE ARE STATED IN TERMS OF CAFFEINE CITRATE.**

2mg caffeine citrate = 1mg caffeine base.

■ **Administration: IV:** bolus (neat, over 3–5 minutes) or as an infusion (over 20 minutes in glucose 5% or NaCl 0.9%).

- **Tablets:** 420mg calcium carbonate and 180mg glycine, <u>providing 168mg (4.2mmol) calcium</u> – Titralac®.
- **Tablets:** 1.25g calcium carbonate, <u>providing 500mg (12.6mmol) calcium</u>; chewable – Calcichew®; effervescent – Cacit®, film-coated – Calcium-500®.
- **Tablets (chewable):** 1.5g calcium carbonate, <u>providing 600mg (15mmol)</u> <u>calcium</u> – Adcal®: 2.5g calcium carbonate, <u>providing 1g (25mmol) calcium</u> – Calcichew®Forte.
- **Tablets:** 300mg calcium carbonate; available as a 'special'.
- **Oral liquid:** 600mg in 5mL; available as a 'special'.

DOSAGE

Route	Age				Frequency (times daily)	Notes
	1 month–2 years	2–12 years		12–18 years		
	<1 year / >1 year	2–6 years	6–12 years			
Oral	120mg / 300mg	300mg	600mg	1.25g	3–4	Initial dose. Subsequently adjusted according to plasma phosphate levels.

NOTES

- Take immediately prior to food to bind phosphate in the food. Titralac® tablets may be chewed, allowed to dissolve in the mouth or swallowed whole, as desired.
- Dose is dependent on serum phosphate level – adjust until this is in normal range and monitor regularly to prevent phosphate depletion syndrome.
- Not suitable as a calcium supplement as only small amounts of calcium are absorbed.
- Plasma calcium should be measured regularly and interpreted in conjunction with plasma protein levels.
- If the patient is also receiving vitamin D, beware hypercalcaemia (measure plasma calcium levels as discussed above).
- Calcichew® and Calcichew® Forte tablets contain aspartame and are unsuitable for patients with phenylketonuria.

■ Licensing varies with the brand of product used. See *Medicines for Children* for details.

■ The oral liquid and the 300mg tablets are available as 'specials' from the Pharmaceutical Production Unit at Guy's and St Thomas' Hospital, London.

Calcium chloride

■ **Injection:** 10% pre-filled syringe (6.8mmol calcium in 10mL).

DOSAGE

Route	Age			Frequency	Notes
	1 month–2 years	2–12 years	12–18 years		
IV	← 0.2mL/kg of the 10% injection →		5–10mL	single dose	Cardiopulmonary resuscitation - ONLY when there is electrolyte disturbance.

NOTES

■ Can cause severe tissue necrosis on extravasation.

■ In cardiac resuscitation, calcium is contra-indicated in the presence of ventricular fibrillation.

■ Licensing varies with the brand of product used. See *Medicines for Children* for details.

■ **Injection:** 10%, 10mL ampoule (contains 2.2mmol calcium in 10mL).

DOSAGE

Route	Age				Frequency	Notes
	birth–1 month	1 month–2 years	2–12 years	12–18 years	(times daily)	
IV bolus over 5–10 minutes	←	0.07mmol/kg (0.3mL/kg of 10% injection)		→	single dose	Hypocalcaemia – urgent correction. Some neonatologists advocate the use of 0.46mmol/kg (2mL/kg of 10% solution) which is a higher dose than that recommended in most UK texts but conforms to practice in the USA.
IV infusion	0.5mmol/kg (0.1mL/kg/hour of 10% injection)	1mmol/kg (0.2mL/kg/hour of 10% injection)	← 8.8mmol/kg total (40mL of the 10% injection)	→	continuous over 24 hours	Hypocalcaemia–maintenance treatment. IV infusion maintenance may be necessary for a few days but the danger of extravasation usually makes oral maintenance preferable. Dilute to at least 0.045mmol/mL with glucose 5% or NaCl 0.9%.
IV bolus	←	0.3mL/kg of 10% solution		→	single dose	Cardiopulmonary resuscitation: only when there is electrolyte disturbance.
IV	1mmol/kg	0.2–1mmol/kg	0.2mmol/kg	5–10mmol total	continuous over 12–24 hours	As part of a parenteral nutrition regimen: quantities are approximate. It depends on individual requirements to maintain normal serum calcium levels.

NOTES

- Not recommended by SC or IM route.

- Monitor plasma calcium carefully.

- Caution in renal impairment.

- Parenteral administration can cause local reactions at injection site and soft tissue calcification.

- Large doses of calcium IV in conjunction with digoxin can cause arrythmias.

- Not licensed in children for the indications stated.

Calcium (oral supplements)

- **Tablets:** ① 600mg calcium gluconate, <u>providing 53.4mg (1.35mmol) calcium.</u> ② 300mg calcium lactate, <u>providing 39mg (1mmol) calcium.</u>
- **Tablets(effervescent):** ① 930mg calcium lactate gluconate, 700mg calcium carbonate and 1.189g anhydrous citric acid, <u>providing 400mg (10mmol) calcium</u> – Sandocal® 400 ② 2.327g calcium lactate gluconate, 1.75 g calcium carbonate and 2.973g anhydrous citric acid, <u>providing 1g (25mmol) calcium</u> – Sandocal® 1000 ③ Calcium gluconate tablets B.P. 1g <u>(1g contains 2.25 mmol of calcium)</u>.
- **Liquid:** each 5mL contains 1.09g calcium glubionate and 727mg calcium lactobionate, <u>providing 108.3mg (2.7mmol) calcium</u> – Calcium Sandoz®.
- **Powder:** each sachet contains 3.3g tricalcium phosphate, <u>providing 1.2g (30mmol) calcium</u> – Ostram®.
- **Granules:** 3.32g hydroxyapatite, <u>providing 712mg (17.8mmol) calcium</u> per sachet – Ossopan®.

DOSAGE

Route	Age				Frequency (times daily)	Notes
	birth-1 month	1 month-2 years	2-12 years	12-18 years		
Oral	← 0.25mmol/kg →		<u>2-4 years</u> 0.25mmol/kg	10mmol	4	
			<u>5-12 years</u> 0.2mmol/kg		4	

NOTES

■ **Administration:** dissolve effervescent tablets in one-third to one-half of a tumbler of water.

In neonates, doses may be mixed with the first (small) part of milk feeds.

■ [L] The liquid is licensed for use in all ages (including neonates). Tablets are licensed for use in adults and children (although the liquid is used <1 year of age). Granules and powder are not licensed for use in children.

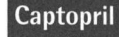

■ **Tablets:** 2mg, 12.5mg, 25mg, 50mg.

■ **Oral liquid:** 5mg in 1mL or may be extemporaneously prepared.

DOSAGE

Route	Age				Frequency (times daily)	Notes
	birth–1 month	1 month–2 years	2–12 years	12–18 years		
Oral	10–50 microgram/kg	◄——— 100 microgram/kg ———►		6.25mg	single dose	Test dose with patient supine. Monitor blood pressure every 15 minutes for 1–2 hours.
	10–50 microgram/kg	◄—100 microgram/kg–2mg/kg—►		–	3	Start at the low dose and titrate up to the maximum if necessary. Use the lowest effective dose. Max dose for <1 month: 2mg/kg/**day**. 1 month–12 years: 6mg/kg/**day**.
	–		–	12.5–50mg	2–3	

NOTES

■ Titrate dose to response.

■ 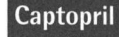 Risk of renal impairment in renovascular disease. Should be avoided in renal artery stenosis or outflow tract obstruction. Patients with renal impairment may respond to smaller or less frequent dosage (titrate dose to response). Removed by dialysis, give 25% of dose after haemodialysis.

■ Not licensed for the treatment of mild to moderate hypertension in children. Licensed in all ages for treatment of congestive heart failure and severe hypertension. The 2mg tablets are available on a named patient basis from Bristol-Myers Squibb and are therefore unlicensed. The 5mg in 1mL oral solution is unlicensed in the UK.

■ 5mg in 1mL oral solution may be imported into the UK via IDIS World Medicines.

■ **Tablets:** 100mg, 200mg, 400mg.
■ **Tablets (modified release):** 200mg, 400mg.
■ **Tablets(chewable):** 100mg, 200mg.

■ **Oral liquid:** 100mg in 5 mL.
■ **Suppositories:** 125mg, 250mg.

DOSAGE

Route	Age				Frequency	Notes
	*birth–1 month	1 month–2 years	2–12 years	12–18 years	(times daily)	
Oral	←	5mg/kg or 2.5mg/kg	→		1 (at night) 2	Starting dose. Increase by 2.5–5mg/kg every 3–7 days until maintenance dose achieved, to reduce incidence of ataxia and drowsiness.
	←		→	100–200mg	1–2	
	←	5mg/kg	→	400–600mg	2 or 3	Usual target maintenance dose. Doses of up to 20mg/kg/day may be needed.
Oral m/r tablets	-	← 5–10mg/kg	→	400–600mg	2	Usual target maintenance dose. (see also non-m/r tablets).
Rectal	-	use approximately 25% more than oral dose (maximum 250mg)			Maximum of 4	Use usually limited to short term replacement of oral therapy.

*Experience with the use of carbamazepine in the neonatal period is very limited.

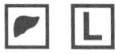

NOTES

■ Dose reduction may be required in advanced liver disease.

■ Auto-induction of carbamazepine metabolism occurs, maximal after 4 weeks; dose may require increasing after initial treatment.

■ Numerous potentially serious interactions with other drugs including other anticonvulsants. Consult product literature for details.

Carbimazole

■ **Tablets:** 5mg, 20mg.

■ **Oral liquid:** manufactured 'special' or may be extemporaneously prepared.

DOSAGE

Route	Age				Frequency	Notes
	birth–1 month	1 month–2 years	2–12 years	12–18 years	(times daily)	
Oral	←	250 microgram/kg	→	10mg	3	Initial dose. Maximum total daily dose 40mg. Administer until euthyroid and then gradually reduce the dose to the minimum (usually given once daily) that sustains normal thyroid function. Alternatively, once euthyroid, continue high dose carbimazole and add levothyroxine 100 microgram/m²/day for

NOTES

- Carbimazole, as methimazole, is excreted into breast milk but this does not preclude breast-feeding as long as neonatal development is closely monitored and the lowest effective dose is used (if possible <15mg daily).

- Contra-indicated in the treatment of hyperthyroidism due to nodular goitre.

- Counsel carer/patient to report symptoms and signs suggestive of infection, especially sore throat or mouth ulceration. A white cell count should be performed and carbimazole stopped if there is evidence of neutropenia.

- 🅛🅔 Licensed for use in children and adults except for the liquid which is available as a 'special' or may be extemporaneously prepared and is therefore unlicensed.

Cefaclor

🅛🅡

- **Capsules:** 250mg, 500mg.
- **Tablet (modified release):** 375mg.

- **Suspension:** 125mg in 5mL, 250mg in 5mL.

DOSAGE

Route	Age			Frequency	Notes
	1 month–2 years	2–12 years	12–18 years	(times daily)	
Oral	<1 year 62.5mg >1 year 125mg	<5 years 125mg >5 years 250mg	250mg	3 3	In severe infections, infections caused by less susceptible organisms doses may be doubled.
Oral m/r tablets	–	–	375mg	2	For the treatment of pneumonia, the dose should be doubled.

Route	Age			Frequency (times daily)	Notes
	1 month–2 years	2–12 years	12–18 years		
Oral for cystic fibrosis patients	<u><1 year</u> 125mg <u>>1 year</u> 250mg	<u><7 years</u> 250mg <u>>7 years</u> 500mg	500mg	3 3	For treatment of asymptomatic *Haemophilus influenzae* carriage or mild exacerbations. 250mg three times daily can be given as 375mg twice daily. 500mg three times daily can be given as 750mg twice daily.

NOTES

- The m/r tablets should be swallowed whole.

- $\boxed{L^Q}$ Not licensed for use <1month of age. The m/r tablets are not licensed for use in children.

Cefadroxil

$\boxed{L}$

- **Capsules:** 500mg.

- **Suspension:** 125mg in 5mL, 250mg in 5mL, 500mg in 5mL.

DOSAGE

Route	Age				Frequency (times daily)	Notes
	birth–1 month	1 month–2 years	2–12 years	12–18 years		
Oral	**DOSE BY WEIGHT** 12.5mg/kg	<u><1 year</u> 12.5mg/kg **DOSE BY AGE** <u>1–2 years</u>	<u>2–6 years</u> 250mg <u>6–12 years</u>	500mg–1g	2	Limited experience of use in premature infants and neonates.

■ **Capsules:** 250mg, 500mg.
■ **Tablets:** 250mg, 500mg.

■ **Syrup:** 125mg in 5mL, 250mg in 5mL, 500mg in 5mL.
■ **Suspension:** 125mg in 5mL, 250mg in 5mL.

DOSAGE

Route	Age			Frequency (times daily)	Notes
	1 month–2 years	2–12 years	12–18 years		
Oral	←	12.5–25mg/kg	→	2	Skin/soft tissue infections, pharyngitis; mild, uncomplicated UTIs. Maximum single dose 1g.
	←	25mg/kg	→	4	Severe infection and otitis media. Maximum single dose 1g.
	62.5-125mg	-	-	2	Other infections.
	-	125–250mg	250–500mg	3	
	←	12.5mg/kg	→	1 (at night)	Urinary tract infection prophylaxis. Maximum dose 125mg.

NOTES

■ C Reduce dose frequency in severe renal failure (creatinine clearance <10mL/min/1.73m²). Dose after haemodialysis.

Tablets: 200mg.

Suspension: 100mg in 5mL; 37.5mL, 75mL.

DOSAGE

Route	Age			Frequency	Notes
	1 month–2 years	2–12 years	12–18.years	(times daily)	
Oral	6 months–1 year 75mg	2–4 years 100mg	200–400mg	1	
	1–2 years 100mg	5–12 years 200mg		1	

NOTES
■ Licensed for use ≥ 6 months of age.

■ **Injection:** 500mg, 1g, 2g vials.

DOSAGE

Newborn infant (birth to 1 month)

Route	Age	Dose	Frequency (times daily)	Notes
IV	<7 days	50mg/kg	2	
	7–21 days	50mg/kg	3	Severe neonatal infections, meningitis.
	>21 days	50mg/kg	3–4	

Child

Route	Age			Frequency (times daily)	Notes
	1 month–2 years	2–12 years	12–18 years		
IV	← 50mg/kg →		1–3g	2	The frequency should be increased to four times daily in meningitis and other severe infections.
IV for cystic fibrosis patients	← 50mg/kg →			3–4	Treatment of severe exacerbations of *Haemophilus influenzae* infection.

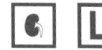

NOTES

■ Dose adjustment in renal impairment: only necessary in severe renal failure (creatinine clearance <10mL/min/1.73m²); give normal dose as loading dose and then half dose at usual frequency. Significantly removed by peritoneal dialysis and haemodialysis, dose after dialysis as for normal renal function.

■ **Administration:** for Claforan® reconstitute with Water for Injections by adding 1.8mL to 500mg vial to give 500mg in 2mL; 3.5mL to 1g vial to give 1g in 4mL; 8.8mL to 2g vial to give 2g in 10mL. For non-proprietary products see manufacturers SPC for details. **IV bolus** - give over 3-5 minutes. **IV infusion** – dilute 4-10 times in glucose 5% or NaCl 0.9% and give over 20-60 minutes.

Cefradine (cephradine)

■ **Capsules:** 250mg, 500mg.

■ **Injection:** 500mg, 1g vials.

■ **Oral liquid:** 250mg in 5mL.

DOSAGE

Route	Age			Frequency	Notes
	1 month–2 years	2–12 years	12–18 years	(times daily)	
Oral	← 12.5mg/kg →		250-500mg	4	Doses may be doubled in severe infection. Maximum of 4g/day.
	or		or		
	25mg/kg		500mg-1g	2	
	← 3mg/kg →		-	1	Prophylaxis for urinary tract infections (if no symptoms

DOSAGE continued

Route	Age			Frequency	Notes
	1 month–2 years	2–12 years	12–18 years	(times daily)	
IV/IM	← 12.5–25mg/kg →		500mg –1g	4	Doses may be doubled in severe infection. Maximum of 8g/**day**.
Oral for cystic fibrosis patients	**DOSE BY WEIGHT**				Continuous anti-staphylococcal therapy. Daily dose can be given in four divided doses if necessary.
	← 12.5–25mg/kg →		-	2	Maximum of 4g/**day**.
	DOSE BY AGE				
	≤1 year 500mg	≤7 years 1g	2g	2	
	>1 year 1g	>7 years 2g		2	

NOTES

■ **Administration: oral:** take after food. **IV:** reconstitute with Water for Injections. Add 4.6mL to the 500mg vial and 9.2mL to the 1g vial to give 100mg in 1mL. Inject slowly over 3-5 minutes. **IV infusion:** reconstitute as for IV injection then dilute with Water for Injections (50mg in 1mL cefradine solutions are approximately isotonic), NaCl 0.9% or glucose 5% and infuse over 30 minutes.

■ ⑥ reduce dose in moderate renal impairment to 50% of a dose every 6 hours or in severe impairment to 25% of a dose every 6 hours.

■ 🄻 Capsules, injection and oral liquid licensed for use in children, except for prophylactic use in Cystic Fibrosis patients. Not licensed for use in neonates.

■ **Injection:** 250mg, 500mg, 1g, 2g, 3g vials.

DOSAGE

Newborn infant

Route	Age		Frequency	Notes
	birth–1 month		(times daily)	
IV	30mg/kg		2	
IV	50mg/kg		2	Dose for treatment of suspected or proven meningitis.

Child

Route	Age			Frequency	Notes
	1 month–2 years	2–12 years	12–18 years	(times daily)	
IV or IM	←	30mg/kg	→	2–3	Doses of up to 50mg/kg given 3 times daily may be used in severe infection to a maximum of 6g per day. Single dose < 1g by IV route only.
IV for cystic fibrosis patients	←	50mg/kg	→	3	Daily dose can be given in two divided doses if necessary. Maximum of 9g per day.
Nebulised for cystic fibrosis patients	←	1g	→	2	Treatment of chronic *Burkholderia cepacia* infection. Dissolve in 3ml of Water for Injections.

Dose adjustment in renal impairment

Creatinine clearance (mL/min/1.73m²)	Dose	Dose frequency
>50	normal	12 hourly
10–50	normal	daily
<10	50%	daily

Haemodialysis: the normal dose should be given after dialysis.
Peritoneal dialysis: 50% of the normal dose should be given initially, then 25-50% of the normal dose once a day. 125-250mg may be added to 2L of dialysis fluid and given in addition to the IV dose.

NOTES
■ **Administration:** displacement value depends on the brand of product used (consult manufacturers literature for details). **IM:** may be reconstituted with 0.5% or 1% lidocaine to concentration 250mg in 1mL. **IV:** dilute to 100mg in 1mL for IV injection; **IV** infusion should be given over 30 minutes.

■ **Injection:** 250mg, 1g, 2g vials.

DOSAGE

Newborn infant

Route	Age	Frequency	Notes
	birth –1 month	(times daily)	
IV	20–50mg/kg	1	Do not exceed 50mg/kg. Infuse over 10–30 minutes (doses of 50mg/kg over at least 60 minutes). Avoid in premature, acidotic or hyperbilirubinaemic neonates.

Child

Route	Age			Frequency	Notes
	1 month–2 years	2–12 years	12–18 years	(times daily)	
IV or IM	←	20–50mg/kg	→	1	Maximum single dose 4g.
IV	←	80mg/kg	→	1	Severe infections. Infuse over 30 minutes.

NOTES

■ Dose adjustment in renal impairment: only necessary in severe renal failure (creatinine clearance <10mL/min/1.73m^2); reduce dose to 50mg/kg or max 2g.

■ **Administration:** may be given by deep IM or IV injection/infusion. **IV:** doses below 50mg/kg may be given by slow injection over 3-5 minutes; higher doses should be infused over at least 30 minutes. Compatible with glucose 5% & 10%, NaCl 0.45% & 0.9% and glucose 4%/NaCl 0.18%. Displacement value is 0.194mL for each 250mg. **IM:** injection may be reconstituted with 1% lidocaine. Manufacturer recommends a concentration of 250mg in 1mL but higher concentrations have been studied and may be more practical, e.g. adding 2.1mL to a 1g vial gives a concentration of 350mg in 1mL. Doses greater than 1g should be divided and injected at more than one site.

Cefuroxime

■ **Tablets:** 125mg, 250mg.
■ **Suspension:** 125mg in 5mL.

■ **Oral powder:** 125mg per sachet.
■ **Injection:** 250mg, 750mg, 1.5g vials

DOSAGE

Newborn infant (birth to 1 month)

Route	Age	Dose	Frequency (times daily)	Notes
IV	<7 days	30mg/kg	2	Treatment of infection.
	>7 days	30mg/kg	3	
	birth–1 month	50mg/kg	2	Severe infection.

Child

Route	Age			Frequency (times daily)	Notes
	1 month–2 years	2–12 years	12–18 years		
IV or IM	←	10–30mg/kg	→	3	20mg/kg/dose is appropriate for most infections. Maximum single dose is 750mg.
	←	50–60mg/kg	→	3–4	Severe infection– reduce the dose, after 3 days or when clinical improvement occurs, to 100mg/kg/day. Maximum single dose is 1.5g.
IV for cystic fibrosis patients	←	50mg/kg	→	3–4	Severe exacerbations of *Haemophilus influenzae* infection. Maximum single dose is 1.5g.
Oral	≥3 months 125mg	250mg	*250mg	2	*May be doubled in severe infection.

Dose adjustment in renal impairment

Creatinine clearance (mL/min/1.73m²)	Dose	Dose frequency
>20	normal	8-12 hourly
10-20	normal	12 hourly
<10	normal	daily

Cefuroxime is significantly removed by haemodialysis. During CAPD, increase the dose interval to 12 hourly.

NOTES

■ **Administration:** may be administered by IM injection, IV injection or IV infusion. Reconstitute with Water for Injections. On reconstitution 250mg powder displaces 0.2mL. **IV infusion:** dilute reconstituted dose with NaCl 0.9% or glucose 5% and give over 30 minutes. **IM:** for IM injection reconstitute with Water for Injection to a final concentration of 250mg in 1mL.

4

Chloral hydrate

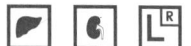

- **Tablets:** chloral betaine 707mg ($\equiv$ chloral hydrate 414mg).
- **Oral solutions:** chloral mixture BP 500mg in 5mL; syrup 500mg in 5mL – available as manufactured 'specials'. Chloral elixir, paediatric, BP 200mg in 5mL – extemporaneously prepared. Elixir 143mg in 5mL.
- **Suppositories:** 25mg, 50mg, 100mg, 250mg, 750mg – available as manufactured 'specials'.

DOSAGE

Indication	Route	Age				Frequency	Notes
		birth–1 month	1 month–2 years	2–12 years	12–18 years	(times daily)	
Sedation for painless procedures	oral/rectal	←	25–50mg/kg	→	1–2g	single dose	Administer about 45–60 minutes prior to the procedure. Single doses up to 100mg/kg have been used prior to scans.
Long-term sedation	oral/rectal	←	20–30mg/kg	→	–	4	Doses up to 50mg/kg administered 4 times daily have been used, but drug accumulation can occur.
Night sedation	oral/rectal	←	30–50mg/kg	→	500mg–1g	single dose (at night)	

NOTES

■ Avoid in cardiac disease, porphyria, respiratory insufficiency and gastritis.

■ Avoid use in moderate to severe renal failure.

■ Avoid use in severe liver disease. May precipitate coma.

■ The tablets are not licensed for use in children. The elixir is not licensed for sedation. The other preparations listed are either manufactured 'specials' or extemporaneously prepared and are therefore unlicensed.

Chloramphenicol

■ **Capsules:** 250mg.
■ **Injection:** 1g vial.
■ **Ear drops:** 5%.

■ **Eye drops:** 0.5%, 5mL and 10mL. Also 0.5mL single use.
■ **Eye ointment:** 1%, 4g.

DOSAGE

Newborn infant (birth to 1 month)

Route	Age	Dose	Frequency (times daily)	Notes
IV bolus	<14 days	12.5mg/kg	2	Monitor levels and adjust dose accordingly.
	>14 days	12.5mg/kg	2–4	

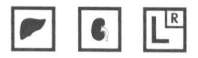

DOSAGE continued

Child

Route	Age			Frequency (times daily)	Notes
	1 month–2 years	2–12 years	12–18 years		
Oral or IV bolus	← 12.5mg/kg →		12.5mg/kg (maximum 1g)	4	Dose may be doubled for severe infection, meningitis, septicaemia; blood levels should be monitored and high doses decreased as soon as clinically indicated.
Oral for cystic fibrosis patients	← 12.5mg/kg →			4	Treatment of chronic *Burkholderia cepacia* infections. Maximum single dose of 1g.
Intra-aural (ear drops)	← 2–3 drops →			2–3	Eye ointment may be used in the ear. (Unlicensed use)
Intra-ocular (eye drops)	← 1 drop →			4–6	A small amount of eye ointment may be used at night in addition to the drops.
Intra-ocular (eye ointment)	← sufficient amount to be massaged into the upper and lower conjunctival sacs →			4	May be used 1–2 hourly in severe infection.

NOTES

■ **Administration: IV:** administer as a bolus IV injection in NaCl 0.9% or glucose 5%.

■ For systemic use, monitor plasma concentration and full blood count. At fifth dose, trough concentration (immediately before dose) to be less than 10mg/L; peak concentration (1 hour after IV or 2 hours after oral) to be 10-20mg/L.

■ Causes bone marrow suppression. This is usually mild and is common when used for more than 7 days. Rarely it is non-dose (concentration)/time related and may then be irreversible.

■ Chloramphenicol is unlikely to be used in breast-feeding mothers. If it is, monitor plasma concentration and full blood count.

■ Grey baby syndrome (abdominal distension, cyanosis, circulatory collapse) may occur in babies with immature hepatic metabolism and/or excessive doses.

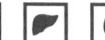

■ **Tablets:** 500mg.

■ **Oral liquid:** 250mg in 5mL.

DOSAGE

Indication	Route	Age				Frequency	Notes
		birth–1 month	1 month–2 years	2–12 years	12–18 years	(times daily)	
Diuresis	Oral	10–17.5mg/kg	<6 months 12.5–17.5mg/kg >6 months 12.5mg/kg	12.5mg/kg	125–500mg	2 2	Doses up to 40mg/kg/day have been used in older children.
Nephrogenic diabetes insipidus	Oral	← 15–17.5mg/kg →			125–500mg	2	
Hyper-insulinism	Oral	← 3.5–5mg/kg →				2	

NOTES

- Contra-indicated in anuria, hypersensitivity to chlorothiazide or other sulphonamide-derived drugs, Addison's disease, hypercalcaemia.

- When creatinine clearance falls below 30mL/min/1.73m², thiazide diuretics become ineffective. Contra-indicated in severe renal failure.

- Use with caution in liver disease; avoid in severe liver disease; minor alterations of fluid and electrolyte balance may precipitate hepatic coma.

- Use with caution in hypokalaemia, asthma, diabetes and in combination with tricyclics, antihypertensives, corticosteroids, NSAIDs, antiarrhythmics, antihistamines, lithium, colestyramine.

- All presentations are unlicensed for use in the UK. The oral liquid is available on a named-patient basis from MSD in the UK; it may also be imported from the USA via IDIS. The tablets may also be imported from the USA via IDIS.

- **Tablets:** 4mg.
- **Oral liquid:** 2mg in 5mL.
- **Injection:** 10mg in 1mL.

DOSAGE

Route	Age			Frequency	Notes
	1 month–2 years	2–12 years	12–18 years	(times daily)	
Oral	1mg	_2–5 years_ 1–2mg _6–12 years_ 2–4mg		2 3 3–4	Maximum total daily doses (oral): 1 month–2 years – 2mg 2–5 years – 6mg 6–12 years – 12mg 12–18 years – 24mg
			4mg	3–4	
IV, IM or SC	_<1 year_ 250 microgram/kg _>1 year_ 2.5–5mg	_2–5 years_ 2.5–5mg _6–12 years_ 5–10mg	10–20mg	single dose	Can be repeated up to 4 times in 24 hours if necessary. Note adult maximum daily dose is 40mg. In anaphylaxis administer IV, as SC or IM rarely acts quicker than oral dosing

NOTES

- **Administration: IV:** dilute with 5-10mL of Water for Injections or NaCl 0.9% and give over 1 minute.

- Licensed for use ≥1 year of age by the oral route. IV, IM, and SC are unlicensed routes of administration in children.

■ **Capsules:** 10mg, 25mg, 50mg, 100mg.
■ **Oral solution:** 100mg in 1mL.

■ **Injection:** 50mg in 1mL; 5mL ampoules.

DOSAGE

Indication	Route	Age			Frequency	Notes
		1 month–2 years	2–12 years	12–18 years	(times daily)	
JIA connective tissue disease, vasculitis and uveitis	Oral	←	1–2mg/kg	→	2	Initial dose. May be increased gradually if required but should not exceed 3mg/kg twice daily.
Organ transplantation	Oral	←	5–7.5mg/kg	→	2	Initial dose given 12 hours before transplantation and continued for 1–2 weeks post-operatively, gradually reducing to a maintenance dose as indicated.
		←	1–3mg/kg	→	2	Maintenance dose.
		←	1.5–4mg/kg	→	2	Lower initial dose if ciclosporin is given with other immunosuppressants as part of triple or quadruple therapy.

DOSAGE continued

Indication	Route	Age			Frequency	Notes
		1 month–2 years	2–12 years	12–18 years	(times daily)	
Bone marrow transplantation (BMT)	Oral	←———	6–7.5mg/kg	———→	2	Initial dose. Start on the day before transplantation. (This dose will vary depending on the type of BMT and protocol).
		←———	6mg/kg	———→	2	Maintenance dose.

If converting from the oral to the intravenous route, give one third the previous oral dose.

NOTES

■ **Administration: oral:** the oral solution should be diluted immediately before administration, preferably with apple juice, orange juice, squash or water, but not with grapefruit juice, as this may alter ciclosporin levels. The measuring device should not come into contact with the diluent and it should not be mixed with water, alcohol or other liquid. **IV:** dilute the concentrated solution 1:20 to 1:100 with NaCl 0.9% or glucose 5% immediately before use, and give over 2-6 hours. The infusion time should not be prolonged beyond 6 hours, as ciclosporin can strip a component from PVC bags and tubing. A fresh solution should be prepared.

■ Doses used in organ transplantation can vary from those indicated depending on individual protocols.

■ Monitor ciclosporin levels, according to local policy.

■ Hepatic or renal function may be impaired with ciclosporin and close monitoring of serum creatinine, urea, electrolyte levels, bilirubin and liver enzymes is required. Dosage should be reduced if necessary.

■ Regular monitoring of blood pressure is required during treatment as ciclosporin may cause hypertension; antihypertensive therapy should be initiated if necessary.

■ Ciclosporin is excreted in breast milk. Women treated with ciclosporin should not breast-feed due to the potential for adverse effects in the infant, including immunosuppression, neutropenia, growth effects and carcinogenesis.

■ Not licensed for use in connective tissue disease, vasculitis and uveitis for any

■ **Tablets:** 200mg, 400mg, 800mg.
■ **Tablets (effervescent):** 400mg.
■ **Oral suspension/syrup:** 200mg in 5mL.

■ **Injection:** 100mg in 1mL; 2mL vial.

DOSAGE

Route	Age				Frequency	Notes
	birth–1 month	1 month–2 years	2–12 years	12–18 years	(times daily)	
Oral or IV infusion	5mg/kg	← 5–10mg/kg →		400mg	4 2–4	Total daily dose may be given in 2 divided doses.

NOTES

■ **Administration: IV:** give IV infusion over at least 10 minutes. Dilute in NaCl 0.9% to give maximum concentration of 10mg in 1mL. May also be given as a continuous infusion. **Oral:** in cystic fibrosis administer 1-2 hours before food.

■ In mild to moderate renal impairment use 75% of the stated doses; in severe impairment use 50% of the dose, at the same time intervals.

■ Reduce dose in hepatic impairment.

■ **Tablets:** 100mg, 250mg, 500mg, 750mg.
■ **Oral liquid:** 250mg in 5mL.

■ **Infusion:** 2mg in 1mL; in NaCl 0.9%, 50ml bottle; in glucose 5%, 100mL, 200mL infusion bags.

DOSAGE

Route	Age				Frequency (times daily)	Notes
	birth–1 month	1 month–2 years	2–12 years	12–18 years		
Oral	←	7.5mg/kg		→	2	Maximum single dose 750mg.
IV	←	5mg/kg		→	2	Maximum single dose 400mg.
Oral for cystic fibrosis patients	–	5–15mg/kg	≤5 years 5–15mg/kg	20mg/kg	2	Treatment for *P. aeruginosa* infection – first isolates or in chronically infected patients with a mild exacerbation.
			≥5 years 20mg/kg		2	
IV for cystic fibrosis patients	–	4–8mg/kg	≤5 years 4–8mg/kg	–	2	Maximum single oral dose is 750mg. Maximum single IV dose is 400mg.
			≥5 years 10mg/kg	10mg/kg	3	

NOTES

■ **Administration: IV:** administer IV infusion over 30–60 minutes; 400mg over 60 minutes

■ In severe renal impairment (creatinine clearance <20mL/min/1.73m²) total daily dosage may be reduced by half, although monitoring serum levels

■ Keep patient well hydrated – crystalluria is a complication.

■  Licensed for use ≥1year of age. Cystic fibrosis dose is only licensed ≥5 years of age.

Clarithromycin

■ **Tablets:** 250mg, 500mg.
■ **Suspension:** 125mg in 5mL, 250mg in 5mL.
■ **Granules:** 250mg/sachet.
■ **Injection:** 500mg vial.

Route	Age				Frequency (times daily)	Notes
	birth–1 month	1 month–2 years	2–12 years	12–18 years		
Oral	DOSE BY WEIGHT					For 5-10 days.
	7.5mg/kg	< 8kg or <1 year 7.5mg/kg	–	–	2	Doses up to 500mg twice daily have been used to treat severe infection.
	–	DOSE BY AGE 1–2 years 62.5mg	3–6 years 125mg	250mg	2	
			7–9 years 187.5mg		2	
			10–12 years 250mg		2	

DOSAGE continued

Route	Age				Frequency (times daily)	Notes
	birth–1 month	1 month–2 years	2–12 years	12–18 years		
Oral for *H.pylori*	–	>1 year 62.5mg	2–6 years- 125mg	500mg	2	Treatment for 14 days with amoxicillin and omeprazole, or metronidazole and omeprazole.
			6–9 years 187.5mg		2	
			9–12 years 250mg		2	
IV infusion	–	← 7.5mg/kg →		500mg	2	Do not give by IV bolus or IM injection.

NOTES

■ **Administration: IV:** reconstitute the 500mg vial with 10mL Water for Injections to give 50mg in 1mL concentration. Then dilute reconstituted dose to 2mg in 1mL with NaCl 0.9% or glucose 5% and give over 1 hour via a large vein.

■ Drug interactions of note: potentiates the effects of theophylline, digoxin, warfarin, carbamazepine. Risk of cardiac arrhythmias with astemizole, cisapride, terfenadine – avoid concurrent use.

■ IV route not licensed for children.

■ **Capsules:** 75mg, 150mg.
■ **Oral liquid:** 75mg in 5mL.

■ **Injection:** 150mg in 1mL; 2mL and 4mL ampoules.
■ **Topical:** 1% as aqueous lotion; 1% in an aqueous alcohol base; 1% gel.

DOSAGE

Route	Age				Frequency (times daily)	Notes
	birth–1 month	1 month–2 years	2–12 years	12–18 years		
Oral	<u><2 weeks</u> 3–6mg/kg	-	-	-	3	
	<u>≥2 weeks</u> 3–6mg/kg	<u><1 year or <10kg</u> 3–6mg/kg	-	-	3-4	In those <1 year or <10kg, the minimum recommended dose is 37.5mg three times a day.
	-	<u>>1 year or >10kg</u> 3–6mg/kg	3–6mg/kg	150–300mg (to a maximum of 450mg in severe infection)	4	
	-	← 5–7mg/kg →			4	Treatment of asymptomatic *S. aureus* isolates or minor exacerbations in cystic fibrosis patients Maximum dose of 600mg four times daily.
IV/IM	5mg/kg	← 5–7mg/kg →		900mg	3	Up to 40mg/kg/day in severe infections or 4.8g/day.

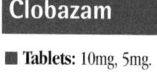

NOTES

■ **Administration: IM:** maximum 600mg (4mL) dose; **IV:** dilute to at least 6mg in 1mL with NaCl 0.9% or glucose 5% and infuse over 10-60 minutes. Avoid rapid administration – maximum rate 20mg/kg over 1 hour.

■ Injection contains benzyl alcohol – associated with fatal Gasping Syndrome in preterm newborns.

■ Discontinue treatment if diarrhoea occurs – may be pseudomembranous colitis.

■ Reduce dose in hepatic impairment; monitor liver function tests.

■ Topical solutions are licensed for use in acne ≥12 years of age; injection licensed for use ≥1 month of age; capsules are licensed for use in children and adults; the oral solution is not a licensed product in the UK (it may be imported into the UK via IDIS).

Clobazam

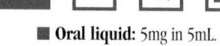

■ **Tablets:** 10mg, 5mg.

■ **Oral liquid:** 5mg in 5mL.

DOSAGE

Route	Age				Frequency	Notes
	birth–1 month	1 month–2 years	2–12 years	12–18 years	(times daily)	
Oral	–	← 125 microgram/kg →		10mg	2	Usual starting dose.
	–	← 250 microgram/kg → (maximum 500 microgram/kg)		10–15mg (maximum 30mg)	2	Usual target maintenance dose. It takes 2–3 weeks to reach the maintenance dose, increasing every 5 days.

NOTES

- ■ 💊 Use reduced dose in severe renal impairment

- ■ 🍃 Caution in severe liver disease; may precipitate coma.

- ■ 🇱 Licensed for use in children ≥3 years of age for epilepsy.
The 5mg tablets may be imported on a named patient basis via IDIS.
The oral liquid is available as a 'special' from North Staffordshire Hospital manufacturing unit. Both preparations are therefore unlicensed.

Clonazepam

- ■ **Tablets:** 500 microgram, 2 mg.
- ■ **Oral liquid:** 500 microgram in 5mL; 2mg in 5mL; 2.5mg in 1mL (100 microgram/drop).

- ■ **Injection:** 1mg in 1mL in solvent; for dilution with 1mL Water for Injections.

DOSAGE

Route	Age				Frequency (times daily)	Notes
	birth–1 month	1 month–2 years	2–12 years	12–18 years		
Oral	–	DOSE BY WEIGHT ← 25 microgram/kg →			1	<u>Starting dose.</u> May be given at night. Higher, divided doses have been used (up to 100 microgram/kg/day).
		DOSE BY AGE <u>≤5 years</u> 250 microgram		1mg	1	
		<u>5–12 years</u> 500 microgram			1	

DOSAGE continued

Route	birth–1 month	1 month–2 years	2–12 years	12–18 years	Frequency (times daily)	Notes
Oral		**DOSE BY WEIGHT** 80 microgram/kg →			3	Usual target maintenance dose.
		DOSE BY AGE				
		<1 year 100–300 microgram			3	The total daily dose may also be divided into 2 or 4 doses.
		1–5 years 300 microgram – 1mg			3	Increase dose from the starting dose every 4 days over 2–4 weeks until satisfactory response, side-effects or maximum dose reached.
		5–12 years 1–2.5mg			3	
		1–2mg			3	
IV bolus over 30 seconds		50 microgram/kg → (maximum 1mg)		1mg	single dose	Status epilepticus. Can be repeated.
IV short infusion	100 microgram/kg				single dose	Can be repeated every 24 hours.
IV infusion		10 microgram/kg/hour (up to 60 microgram/kg/hour has been given)			continuous	Bolus loading dose is usually administered first. Adjust to response.

NOTES

■ **Administration: IV:** mix active substance with diluent before IV administration. IV bolus over at least 30 seconds, short infusion of 100 microgram in 1ml diluent preferred in neonates. May be infused neat into suitably placed cannula, dilution preferred in glucose 5%, glucose 10%, NaCl 0.9% or glucose/saline, maximum concentration 12mg/litre. Dilutions should be changed every 12 hours. Clonazepam can be absorbed onto PVC. It is therefore recommended that glass containers be used or, if PVC infusion bags are used, that the mixture is infused straight-away over a period of no longer than 2 hours. In practice, problems do not seem to have been encountered with PVC-free syringes e.g. polypropelene plastic syringes.

- ■ Use reduced dose in severe renal impairment.
- ■ Use with caution in severe liver disease; may precipitate coma.
- ■ Licensed for use in all ages except for the oral liquid preparations which are not licensed products.
- ■ Both oral liquid preparations are available as 'specials' from Rosemont. The oral drops may be imported via IDIS.

Co-amoxiclav (amoxicillin and clavulanic acid)

- ■ **Tablets:** 375mg (250/125), 625mg (500/125).
- ■ **Tablets (dispersible):** 375mg (250/125).
- ■ **Suspension:** 125/31 in 5mL, 250/62 in 5mL, 400/57 in 5mL.
- ■ **Injection:** 600mg (500/100), 1.2g (1000/200) vials.

DOSAGE

Newborn infant

Route	Age		Frequency (times daily)	Notes
	<7 days	>7 days		
Oral	← 0.25mL/kg (of the 125/31 suspension) →		3	
IV	30mg/kg	-	2	Dosage is based on co-amoxiclav content.
	-	30mg/kg	3	

Child

Route	Age			Frequency	Notes
	1 month-2 years	2-12 years	12-18 years	(times daily)	
Oral	≤1 year 0.25mL/kg of the 125/31 suspension	2-6 years 5mL of the 125/31 suspension	1 tablet (250/125)	3	Doses may be doubled in severe infections with the suspensions. In severe infections with the tablet give 1 tablet (500/125) per dose.
	>1 year 5mL of the 125/31 suspension	7-12 years 5mL of the 250/62 suspension		3	
Oral (400/57 suspension)	2 months-2 years 0.15mL/kg	2-6 years 2.5mL	-	2	Mild to moderate infection.
		7-12 years 5mL	-	2	
	2 months-2 years 0.3mL/kg	2-6 years 5mL	-	2	Severe infection.
		7-12 years 10mL	-	2	
IV	← 30mg/kg →		1.2g	3	Dosage is based on co-amoxiclav content. Over 3 months of age the dose frequency can be increased to 4 times

Dose adjustment in renal impairment

Creatinine clearance (mL/min/1.73m²)	Dose	Dose frequency
10-30	Oral – normal	12 hourly
	IV – normal initial dose then 50%	12 hourly
<10	Oral – 50%	12 hourly
	IV – normal initial dose then 50%	daily

NOTES

- **Administration: IV:** reconstitute with Water for Injections: 600mg vial with 10mL (final volume 10.5mL); 1.2g with 20mL (final volume 20.9mL). Give as a slow IV injection over 3-4 minutes within 20 minutes of reconstitution or infuse over 30-40 minutes completing within 4 hours of reconstitution.

- Compatible with NaCl 0.9% and can be diluted to 5 times its volume. Unstable in glucose solutions.

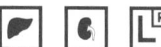

■ **Tablets:** 15mg, 30mg, 60mg.
■ **Syrup:** 25mg in 5mL; codeine linctus BP (codeine phosphate 15mg in 5mL).

■ **Injection:** 60mg in 1mL (controlled drug).
■ **Suppositories:** 1mg, 2mg, 3mg, 6mg; available as manufactured 'specials'.

DOSAGE

Route	Age				Frequency (times daily)	Notes
	birth–1 month	1 month–2 years	2–12 years	12–18 years		
Oral Rectal IM/SC	← 500 microgram–1mg/kg →			30–60mg	4–6 (maximum daily dose 240mg)	Repeated doses increase the risk of respiratory depression. Avoid IM injections if possible. Use IM/SC cannula placed while under GA or topical LA. Codeine phosphate can cause severe constipation so prophylactic laxatives should always be prescribed.

NOTES
■ 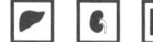 Avoid in renal or hepatic impairment.

■ Avoid in acute respiratory depression or paralytic ileus.

■ Naloxone may be used as an antidote.

■ Not licensed for use <1 year of age. Suppositories are not licensed preparations.

There are many topical corticosteroid and combination preparations available, some of which are listed below. For full details refer to *Medicines for Children*.

DOSAGE

Corticosteroid preparations

Drug Name	Presentation	Potency
Hydrocortisone	Cream, ointment; 0.5%, 1%.	Mild
Clobetasone butyrate	Cream, ointment; 0.05%.	Moderate
Betamethasone esters	Cream, ointment; 0.025%.	Moderate
	Cream, ointment, lotion; 0.05%.	Potent
	Cream, ointment, scalp application, lotion, foam; 0.1%.	Potent
Clobetasol propionate	Cream, ointment, scalp application, 0.05%.	Very potent

Initial treatment should usually be with hydrocortisone, particularly in infants less than 12 months. Apply sparingly to the affected areas once or twice a day.

NOTES

■ All preparations are licensed for use> 1 year of age.

96 Co-trimoxazole

A 5:1 mixture of two antibiotics, sulphamethoxazole and trimethoprim.
(Sulphamethoxazole = S; Trimethoprim = T)

- **Tablets (dispersible):** 400mg S/80mg T.
- **Tablets:** 800mg S/160mg T.
- **Adult suspension:** 400mg S/80mg T in each 5ml.
- **Paediatric suspension:** 200mg S/40mg T in each 5ml.
- **Intravenous infusion:** 400mg S/80mg T in each 5ml ampoule.

DOSAGE

Indication	Route	Age 1 month–2 years	Age 2–12 years	Age 12–18 years	Frequency (times daily)	Notes
Systemic infection	Oral	DOSE BY WEIGHT 24mg/kg →	→	-	2	Dose may be doubled in severe infection.
		DOSE BY AGE 6 weeks–5 months 120mg / 6 months–2 years 240mg	2–5 years 240mg / 6–12 years 480mg	960mg	2	
	IV	18–27mg/kg →	→	→	2	The higher dose stated is that used in severe infection.
Prophylaxis of urinary tract infection	Oral	12mg/kg →	→	480mg	1 (at night)	Only if bacterial sensitivities indicate and there is good reason to prefer co-trimoxazole to a single antibiotic. Maximum single dose 1.44g.

DOSAGE continued

Indication	Route	Age			Frequency (times daily)	Notes
		1 month–2 years	2–12 years	12–18 years		
Pneumocystis carinii treatment	Oral/ IV	←	60mg/kg or	→	2	For 10–14 days. Oral route is preferred unless nausea is severe.
		←	30mg/kg	→	4	
Pneumocystis carinii prophylaxis	Oral	← body surface area 0.5–0.75m² 240mg →		960mg	2	On two or three days of the week e.g. Mondays, Wednesdays and Fridays or Mondays and Tuesdays depending or protocol.
		← body surface area 0.76–1.0m² 360mg →			2	
		← body surface area>1m² 480mg →			2	

Dosage is indicated in terms of the total amount of drug in milligrams, e.g. 24mg/kg is 20mg/kg sulphamethoxazole and 4mg/kg trimethoprim.

Dose adjustment in renal impairment

Creatinine clearance (mL/min/1.73m²)	Dosage
>30	Normal dose
15-30	Normal dose for 3 days then half the dose
<15	Avoid unless haemodialysis is available, and then give half the normal dose.

Co-trimoxazole is <u>not</u> removed by peritoneal dialysis.

NOTES

- **Administration: oral:** take with food or drink to minimise the possibility of gastrointestinal disturbances. **IV infusion:** must be diluted before administration and dilution should be carried out immediately before use. Dilute 1 in 25 with NaCl 0.9% or glucose 5%. In severely fluid restricted patients dilute 1 in 10 in glucose 5%. Dilution to less than 1 in 10 is not possible as the propylene glycol precipitates out. After adding co-trimoxazole for infusion to the infusion solution shake thoroughly to ensure complete mixing. If visible turbidity or crystallisation appears at any time before or during an infusion, the mixture should be discarded. Infuse over 60-90 minutes. In severe fluid restriction can be given undiluted via the central route.

- Not licensed for use <6 weeks of age.

- The use of co-trimoxazole is not generally recommended under 6 weeks of age, but some neonatologists feel that there is no specific reason for this caution other than the concerns relating to G6PD deficiency. If it is used in newborn infants, it is given in the same dosage as for 6 weeks – 5 months (see table) but trimethoprim on its own is now normally preferred to co-trimoxazole.

Tablets: 50mg.

Injection: (as lactate) 50mg in 1mL, 1mL ampoule.

Oral liquid: may be extemporaneously prepared, manufactured 'special'.

Suppositories: 12.5mg, 25mg, 50mg and 100mg – manufactured 'special'.

DOSAGE

Route	Age			Frequency	Notes
	1 month–2 years	2–12 years	12–18 years	(times daily)	
Oral/IV bolus	← DOSE BY WEIGHT →			3	Maximum single dose:
	500 microgram/kg - 1mg/kg				<6 years 25mg
Oral/rectal		DOSE BY AGE			> 6 years 50mg.
	-	2-5 years	12-18 years		
		12.5mg	50mg	3	
		6-12 years			
		25mg		3	
IV or SC infusion	3mg/kg	2-5 years	150mg	continuous infusion over 24 hours	Can be combined with other drugs. Check compatibility.
		50mg			
		6-12 years			
		75mg			

NOTES

■ **Administration: IV:** by slow IV injection over 3-5 minutes. May be diluted if required to a maximum 1:1 dilution with Water for Injections only. Can be given as a continuous IV infusion. **Oral:** tablets may be crushed and dispersed in water. **SC:** occasionally associated with irritation at site of continuous SC infusion. If affected consider increasing the dilution of drug in the infusion or adding hyaluronidase or low dose hydrocortisone to the syringe. Do not mix with any solution containing chloride ions as this will lead to precipitate formation.

■ Use with caution in hepatic disease (may induce coma).

■ Licensed ≥6 years of age, for all indications. Suppositories are 'specials' and as such are unlicensed. Oral liquid is a 'special' or may be extemporaneously prepared and as such is unlicensed.

■ Suspension and suppositories available from Martindale Pharmaceuticals and Aurum Pharmaceuticals Ltd.

■ **Tablets:** 50mg.
■ **Oral liquid:** manufactured 'special' or may be extemporaneously prepared.

■ **Injection:** 200mg, 500mg, 1g vials.

DOSAGE

Treatment of malignant disease

Wide variation in dosage. Dose interval and cumulative dose vary depending on protocol.
** Always consult the current treatment protocol for details of dosage and scheduling. **

Other indications

Indication	Route	Age			Frequency	Notes
		1 month-2 years	2-12 years	12-18 years		
Nephrotic syndrome	Oral	←	2–3mg/kg	→	once daily in the morning	For up to 12 weeks.
Vasculitis SLE	IV	←	500mg-1g/m²	→	once monthly	More frequent administration may be necessary in severe disease.

NOTES

■ **Administration:** IV: by slow IV bolus into established IV line; by IV infusion in glucose 5%, NaCl 0.9% or glucose/saline infusion. In order to prevent urothelial toxicity, hydration and mesna are required, particularly with higher daily doses of the drug. The manufacturers recommend concurrent mesna administration for daily doses of cyclophosphamide in excess of 10mg/kg (300mg/m²). In paediatric clinical practice, mesna is not required until higher daily, or cumulative doses, per course are exceeded, providing adequate hydration and micturition can be maintained, although in rheumatological practice, mesna is usually given whatever the dose.

Daily cyclophosphamide dose <10mg/kg (<300mg/m²)
No mesna. Maintain fluid intake, encourage micturition.

Daily, or total course cyclophosphamide dose 300mg/m² - 1g/m²
No mesna. IV hydration with glucose/saline at 3L/m²/24 hours commencing with first cyclophosphamide dose and continuing for at least 6 hours after last cyclophosphamide dose.

Daily, or total course cyclophosphamide dose >1g/m²
IV hydration with glucose/saline containing mesna at at 3L/m²/24 hours. Mesna doses vary but in practice doses greater than 100% (mg:mg) of the prescribed daily cyclophosphamide dose are used. Start hydration 3 hours before first cyclophosphamide dose and continue for at least 12 hours after the last cyclophosphamide dose.

■ Oral liquid available from Nova laboratories. Various strengths can be manufactured with an expiry date of 14 days.

■ Contra-indicated in concurrent acute urinary tract infection or urothelial damage following previous cytotoxic chemotherapy or pelvic irradiation.

■ Full blood count and assessment of renal and hepatic function should be obtained prior to each course of therapy.

■ Vasculitis, SLE, nephrotic syndrome are not licensed indications in any age group.

■**Injection:** 2500 units in 1mL; 4mL ampoule.

■**Injection:** 10,000 units in 1mL; 1mL graduated syringe and 1mL ampoule.

■**Injection:** 12,500 units in 1mL; 2500 units in 0.2mL syringe.

■**Injection:** 25,000 units in 1mL; 5000 units in 0.2mL, 7500 units in 0.3mL, 10,000 units in 0.4mL, 12,500 units in 0.5mL, 15,000 units in 0.6mL and 18,000 units in 0.72mL syringe, 4mL vial.

DOSAGE

Indication	Route	Age				Frequency (times daily)	Notes
		birth– 1 month	1 month– 2 years	2–12 years	12–18 years		
Treatment dose	SC	←	100 units/kg	→	-	2	
			-		200 units/kg	1	The single daily dose should not exceed 18,000 units.
Treatment dose if increased risk of bleeding	SC		-		100 units/kg	2	
Prophylaxis dose	SC	←	100 units/kg	→	2500-5000 units	1	

Experience is very limited in children and even more limited in neonates.

NOTES

- Patients with severely disturbed hepatic function may need a reduction in dosage and should be monitored accordingly.

- The half-life is prolonged in uraemic patients as dalteparin sodium is eliminated primarily through the kidneys.

- When considered necessary, it is recommended that the antithrombotic effect be monitored by analysing anti-Factor Xa activity using a suitable assay. This is because dalteparin has only a moderate prolonging effect on clotting time assays such as APTT or thrombin time.

- As different low molecular weight heparins may not be equivalent, alternative products should not be substituted during a course of treatment.

Desmopressin

 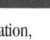

- **Nasal spray:** 10 microgram per actuation; 2.5 microgram per actuation, 150 microgram per actuation.
- **Intranasal solution:** 100 microgram in 1mL.

- **Tablets:** 100 microgram, 200 microgram.
- **Injection:** 4 microgram in 1mL.

DOSAGE

Indication	Route	Age				Frequency (times daily)	Notes
		birth–1 month	1 month–2 years	2–12 years	12–18 years		
Established diabetes insipidus	Intranasal	1.25-5 microgram	2.5-5 microgram	5-20 microgram	10-20 microgram	1-2	Individual dose titration required. A trial of monitored treatment may be used as a diagnostic test.
	Oral	5 microgram	5-50 microgram	50-200 microgram	50-300 microgram	3	
Nocturnal enuresis	Intranasal	–	–	≥5 years ←——— 20 microgram ———→		1 (at night)	Half the total dose is given into each nostril. Increase if necessary to a maximum of 40 microgram (20 microgram in each nostril) at night. Reassess after 3 months by stopping treatment for at least 1 week.
	Oral	–	–	≥5 years ←——200 microgram——→		1 (at night)	Increase if necessary to a maximum of 400 microgram at night. Reassess after 3 months by stopping treatment for at least 1 week.

DOSAGE continued

Indication	Route	Age				Frequency	Notes
		birth– 1 month	1 month– 2 years	2–12 years	12–18 years	(times daily)	
Mild - moderate haemophilia and von Willebrand disease	IV	-	←	>1 year 300 nanogram/kg	→	single dose	Discuss with haematologist. Dilute in 30-50mL NaCl 0.9% and give over 20 minutes, immediately before surgery. Can be repeated after 12 hours, only if no tachycardia
	Intranasal	-	←	4 microgram/kg	→	single dose	If used preoperatively use 2 hours prior to procedures.

NOTES

■ **Administration: oral:** tablets are scored, and may be halved or crushed. **Intranasal:** children requiring <10 microgram as a dose should use the dropper bottle with catheter for nasal administration or the 2.5 microgram per actuation nasal spray which is available on a named-patient basis from the manufacturers. **IV:** when used for haemophilia or von Willebrand disease dilute in 30-50 mL NaCl 0.9%. It should not be diluted in patients with diabetes insipidus requiring a dose of 4 micrograms or less.

■ **In treating diabetes insipidus monitor the effects carefully and adjust the dosage accordingly.**

■ 🄻ᴿ The 10 microgram per actuation intranasal spray and the Desmotabs® brand of 200 microgram tablets are licensed for use in primary nocturnal enuresis in patients ≥5 years of age. The intranasal solution, the

10 microgram per actuation intranasal spray and the injection are licensed for the diagnosis and treatment of vasopressin-sensitive cranial diabetes insipidus in all ages. The DDAVP® brand of tablets (100 and 200 microgram) are licensed for the treatment of vasopressin-sensitive cranial diabetes insipidus in all ages. Only the injection is licensed for use in haemophilia and von Willebrands disease.

■ Contra-indicated in cardiac insufficiency and other conditions requiring treatment with diuretic agents. The diagnosis of a psychogenic polydipsia should be excluded prior to treatment. Avoid water load (including swallowing during swimming). Stop if intercurrent diarrhoea/vomiting. Caution in cardiovascular disease and cystic fibrosis.

■ C Use with great caution in renal disease.

Dexamethasone

■ **Tablets:** 500 microgram, 2mg.
■ **Oral solution:** 2mg in 5mL, 500 microgram in 5mL.
■ **Injection:** dexamethasone sodium phosphate 5mg in 1mL, 1mL ampoule, 2mL vial.

■ **Injection:** dexamethasone phosphate 4mg in 1mL, 1mL ampoule, 2mL vial.

DOSAGE

NOTE: 1mg of dexamethasone base ≡ 1.2mg of dexamethasone phosphate ≡ 1.3mg of dexamethasone sodium phosphate. Prescribe in terms of **dexamethasone base**, with the exception of the treatment of cerebral oedema.

<u>Fetal lung maturation: given to the mother</u>
IM dosage: 12mg dexamethasone base, repeated once after 24 hours if the risk of preterm delivery remains.
Or can be given orally. **Oral dosage:** 6mg dexamethasone base orally twice daily for four doses.

<u>Chronic Lung Damage ('bronchopulmonary dysplasia' or BPD)</u>
The optimal regimen has not yet been determined. Regimens commonly used include:
250 microgram/kg dexamethasone base orally or IV twice daily for 3 days – regimen repeated once every ten days until the baby is no longer oxygen dependent.
500 microgram/kg dexamethasone base orally or IV once daily for 3 days, then progressively reduced over a 6 week period to 100 microgram/kg on alternate days during the last week.

<u>Post intubation laryngeal oedema</u>
Three 200 microgram/kg doses of **dexamethasone base** orally or IV 8 hourly, starting 4 hours before extubation.

<u>Chemotherapy regimes</u>
Always follow the dosage recommended in the chemotherapy protocol.

Cerebral oedema : High dose IV schedule (dose in terms of **dexamethasone phosphate**).

	Children <35kg	Children >35kg
Initial dose	20mg	24mg
1st–3rd day	4mg every 3 hours	4mg every 2 hours
4th day	4mg every 6 hours	4mg every 4 hours
5–8th day	2mg every 6 hours	4mg every 6 hours
Thereafter	decrease by daily reduction of 1mg	decrease by daily reduction of 2mg

Indication	Route	Age			Frequency (times daily)	Notes
		1 month–2 years	2–12 years	12–18 years		
Croup	Oral	← 150 microgram/kg → or ← 600 microgram/kg →		–	2 single dose	No definitive standard dose has been agreed in the UK. Suggested maximum single dose of 12mg.
Anti-emetic	IV/oral	<1 year 250 microgram–1mg 1–2 years 1–2mg	2–5 years 1–2mg 6–12 years 2–4mg	4mg	3 3	Give IV doses with chemotherapy, then give IV or orally until 48 hours after chemotherapy.

DOSAGE continued

Indication	Route	Age			Frequency (times daily)	Notes
		1 month– 2 years	2–12 years	12–18 years		
Headache associated with raised intracranial pressure	IV/oral	← 250 microgram/kg →			2	For 5 days; then reduce if possible to 62.5–125 microgram/kg twice daily.
Short course to relieve symptoms of brain tumour	IV/oral	← 125–500 microgram/kg →			2	Can also be used to reduce oedema around tumours compressing nerves.
Replacement	IV/oral	← 250 –500 microgram/m² →			2	

NOTES

■ **Administration: IV:** give as a bolus over 3-5 minutes, neat or diluted in NaCl 0.9% or glucose 5%.

■ Prescribe as dexamethasone base.

■ 1mg dexamethasone base ≡ 1.2mg dexamethasone phosphate ≡ 1.3mg dexamethasone sodium phosphate.

■ ⃞ BPD, foetal lung maturation, croup and anti-emetic use are not licensed indications in children. The 500microgram in 5mL oral solution is an

Diamorphine hydrochloride (controlled drug)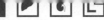

■ **Tablets:** 10mg.
■ **Injection:** 5mg, 10mg, 30mg, 100mg, 500mg ampoules.

■ **Oral solution:** may be extemporaneously prepared.

DOSAGE
Newborn infant - ventilated

Route	Age	Frequency	Notes
	birth–1 month		
Start IV infusion (over 30 minutes)	50 microgram/kg	single dose	Loading dose. Infant ventilated.
IV infusion	15 microgram/kg/hour	continuous	Maintenance dose. Infant ventilated.

The above doses have been used to provide analgesia and to improve synchrony during mechanical ventilation.
Infusions of 2.5–7 microgram/kg/hour have been used in non-ventilated newborn infants.

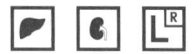

Child

Route	Age			Frequency	Notes
	1 month–2 years	2–12 years	12–18 years		
Oral	← 100–200 microgram/kg →		10mg	single dose	Repeat every 4 hours as necessary.
IV bolus	1–3 months 20 microgram/kg	-	-	single dose	Repeat every 6 hours as necessary.
	3–6 months 25–50 microgram/kg	-	-	single dose	Repeat every 6 hours as necessary.
	6–12 months 75 microgram/kg	-	-	single dose	Repeat every 4 hours as necessary.
	>12 months ← 75–100 microgram/kg →		2.5–5mg	single dose	Repeat every 4 hours as necessary.
IV infusion	← 12.5– 25 microgram/kg/hour →		-	continuous	
SC infusion	← 20–100 microgram/kg/hour →			continuous	
Extradural injection	← 25–50 microgram/kg/dose →			single dose	
SC/IM injection	-	-	5mg	single dose	Repeat every 4 hours as necessary. Use with caution if poor peripheral perfusion. Avoid IM injections if possible. Use SC/IM cannula placed while under GA or topical LA

NOTES

■ **Administration: SC:** reconstitute 5-100mg ampoules with 1mL Water for Injections and the 500mg ampoule with 2mL; for SC infusion dilute reconstituted ampoules with Water for Injections or for concentrations up to 40mg per mL NaCl 0.9% can be used but precipitation is more likely. Inspect solutions carefully for signs of precipitation after reconstitution and during administration. **IV infusion:** glucose 5% is the preferred diluent.

■ Avoid in acute respiratory depression and paralytic ileus.

■ Use with caution in raised intra-cranial pressure, head injury or biliary colic.

■ Naloxone may be required as an antidote.

■ Avoid or reduce dose in liver disease - may precipitate coma.

■ In severe renal impairment give 50-75% of dose.

■ In children, diamorphine injection is only licensed for the treatment of those who are terminally ill; use for other indications and in newborn infants is unlicensed. Tablets are not licensed for use in children.

Diazepam

■ **Tablets:** 2mg, 5mg, 10mg.
■ **Oral liquid:** 2mg in 5mL, 5mg in 5mL.
■ **Injection (solution):** 5mg in 1mL; 2mL ampoule.
■ **Injection (emulsion):** 5mg in 1mL; 2mL ampoule.

■ **Rectal tubes:** 2mg in 1mL, 1.25mL (2.5mg tube), 2.5mL (5mg tube); 4mg in 1mL, 2.5mL (10mg tube).
■ **Suppositories:** 10mg.

DOSAGE

Route	Indication	birth–1 month	1 month–2 years	2–12 years	12–18 years	Frequency (times daily)	Notes
Oral	Pre-medication	–	DOSE BY WEIGHT ≤1 year 250 microgram/kg DOSE BY AGE >1 year 2.5mg	<5 years 2.5mg >5 years 5mg	10mg	single dose	
						single dose	
IV	Sedation prior to procedures, procedures, calming during procedures	–	← 100–200 microgram/kg →			single dose	IV only to be given by a trained anaesthetist or intensivist and very slow titration against symptoms or level of consciousness to a maximum of: 5mg <12 years 10–20mg >12 years. Orally give 45–60 minutes before procedure.
Oral		–	← 200–300 microgram/kg →			single dose	
Rectal		–	>1 year 5mg	2–3 years 5mg >3 years 5–10mg	10mg	single dose	

DOSAGE continued

Indication	Route	Age				Frequency	Notes
		birth– 1 month	1 month– 2 years	2–12 years	12–18 years	(times daily)	
Status epilepticus	IV bolus	← 300-400 microgram/kg →			10–20mg	single dose	Lorazepam is first choice benzodiazepine IV (see guidance section in *Medicines for Children*).
	IV infusion	50 microgram /kg/hour (maximum 300 microgram /kg/hour)	←100 microgram/kg/hour→ (maximum usually 125 micrograms/kg/hour but doses of up to a maximum of 400 microgram/kg/hour have been used in PICU)		125 microgram/ kg/hour	continuous	Diazepam IV is an alternative. Repeat diazepam IV bolus after 10 minutes if necessary. IV infusion: start at the lower dose, increasing if necessary to the maximum as indicated.
	Rectal	1.25–2.5mg	5mg	5–10mg	10mg	single dose	If needed, repeat after 5 minutes.

NOTES

- ▣ tablets and oral liquid licensed for use in children for night terrors, somnambulism, pre-medication, management of cerebral spasticity and control of muscle spasm in tetanus. Injection licensed in children for status epilepticus, febrile convulsions, convulsions due to poisoning and for pre-medication. The rectal tubes are licensed for use in children > 1 year of age for acute severe anxiety and agitation, epileptic and febrile convulsions, tetanus and sedation for procedures.

- ▣ In severe renal impairment use reduced doses (increased cerebral sensitivity). Dose reduction is not necessary in mild to moderate renal impairment.

- ▣ Dose reduction is not necessary in liver disease. Caution in severe liver disease; may precipitate coma.

- Parenteral and rectal use can depress respiration.

116 Diazoxide

R | 🫘

■ **Tablets:** 50mg.
■ **Oral liquid:** may be extemporaneously prepared.
■ **Injection:** 15mg in 1mL, 20mL ampoule.

DOSAGE

Indication	Route	Age				Frequency (times daily)	Notes
		birth–1 month	1 month–2 years	2–12 years	12–18 years		
Intractable hypo-glycaemia	Oral	← 1.7–5mg/kg →				3	Initial dose – to establish response. Thereafter, dose can be increased as necessary. Usual maximum dose is 15mg/kg/day although up to 20mg/kg/day has been used in hyperinsulinism of infancy.
Resistant hypertension	Oral	← 1.7mg/kg →				3	
Severe hypertension	IV bolus	–	← 1–3mg/kg → (maximum of 150mg)			single dose	Repeat after 5–15 minutes if necessary. Monitor blood pressure closely. Maximum 4 doses in 24 hours.

NOTES

■ Seek expert advice before prescribing.

■ **Administration: IV:** give as a rapid injection over 30 seconds or less. Never give by the IM or SC routes as it is very irritant.

■ Retention of sodium and water may occur.

■ Caution in patients with severe renal impairment.

■ Monitor white cell and platelet count regularly when used over a prolonged period.

■ May cause hypertrichosis with long term use.

■ Tablets are licensed for use in both children and adults. Oral liquid can be prepared from powder which is available from Medeva Pharma Ltd on named patient basis, and is therefore an unlicensed product.

Diclofenac sodium

■ **Tablets (dispersible):** 10mg ('special'), 50mg.
■ **Tablets (enteric coated):** 25mg, 50mg.
■ **Tablets (modified release):** 75mg, 100mg.
■ **Capsules (modified release):** 75mg, 100mg.

■ **Capsule:** (25mg enteric coated; 50mg modified release).
■ **Suppositories:** 12.5mg, 25mg, 50mg, 100mg.
■ **Injection:** 25mg in 1mL, 3mL ampoule.
■ **Gel:** 1%.

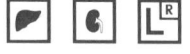

DOSAGE

Route	Age			Frequency (times daily)	Notes
	1 month–2 years	2–12 years	12–18 years		
Oral/rectal	<u><6 months</u> Not recommended <u>>6 months</u> 300 microgram–1mg/kg	← 300 microgram/kg–1mg/kg →		3	Up to a maximum of 150mg/day.
IM/IV	<u><6 months</u> Not recommended <u>>6 months</u> 300 microgram–1mg/kg	← 300 microgram/kg–1mg/kg →		1–2	Up to a maximum of 150mg/day, and for a maximum of 2 days.
Topical	Not recommended	← Small amount →		3–4	

NOTES

■ **Administration: IV:** do not administer as an IV bolus injection. 75mg of diclofenac should be diluted in 100-500mL of either NaCl 0.9% or glucose 5%. These solutions must first be buffered with sodium bicarbonate solution (0.5mL of 8.4% or 1mL of 4.2%). The dose should be infused over 30 minutes to 2 hours. IV therapy should not continue for more than 2 days.

■ Use with caution in patients with renal impairment, or severe liver impairment.

- Avoid in patients with active peptic ulcer disease and in patients who have previously shown hypersensitivity reactions (asthma, rhinitis, urticaria) to aspirin or other NSAIDs.

- The IV route is contra-indicated with concurrent NSAID or anticoagulant use or a history of haemorrhagic diathesis.

- L^R All the 25mg enteric coated tablets and the 12.5mg and 25mg

suppositories are licensed for use in juvenile idiopathic arthritis >1 year of age at a dose of 1–3mg/kg/day in divided doses. Volraman® 50mg EC tablets are the only 50mg tablets licensed for this age group for the same dose and indication. All other preparations containing ≥50mg diclofenac are not licensed for use in children. 10mg dispersible tablets are a 'special' and as such are unlicensed.

- 10mg dispersible tablets are available from Special Products Limited.

Digoxin

- **Tablets:** 62.5, 125, 250 microgram.
- **Elixir:** 50 microgram in 1mL.

- **Injection:** 250 microgram in 1mL, 2mL ampoule; 100 microgram in 1mL, available as a 'special'.

DOSAGE

The doses stated are for patients who have not received cardiac glycosides in the preceding two weeks. If cardiac glycosides have been given in the two weeks preceding commencement, it should be anticipated that optimum loading doses will be less than those stated (levels should be checked before loading).

The dosage schedules are meant as guidelines and careful clinical observation and monitoring of serum digoxin levels should be used as a basis for adjustment of dosage.

In myocarditis, halve the loading and maintenance doses, as the myocardium is more sensitive to cardiac glycosides.

Check the doses carefully because an overdose can cause death.

Maintenance dose should start 12 hours after loading is complete.

* >10 years use doses at the lower end of the range in early adolescence and/or in underweight children.

LOADING DOSE

The loading dose (IV or oral) should be administered in divided doses over 12 hours. Give half the total loading dose immediately, a quarter of the total loading dose after 6 hours and the remainder after a further 6 hours, assessing the clinical response before giving each additional dose. Each IV dose should be given by slow IV bolus over 10 minutes.

Intravenous loading dose

Age	Pre-term newborn infant <1.5kg	Pre-term newborn infant 1.5-2.5kg	Newborn infant to 2 years	2 to 5 years	5 to 10 years	*>10 years
Dose	10 microgram/kg over 10 minutes	15 microgram/kg over 10 minutes	← 17.5 microgram/kg over 10 minutes →		12.5 microgram/kg over 10 minutes (max 250 microgram)	250–500 microgram over 10 minutes
	then after 6 hours 5 microgram/kg over 10 minutes	then after 6 hours 7.5 microgram/kg over 10 minutes	then after 6 hours ← 8.75 microgram/kg over 10 minutes →		then after 6 hours 6.25 microgram/kg over 10 minutes (max 125 microgram)	then after 6 hours 125–250 microgram over 10 minutes
	then after a further 6 hours 5 microgram/kg over 10 minutes	then after a further 6 hours 7.5 microgram/kg over 10 minutes	then after a further 6 hours ← 8.75 microgram/kg over 10 minutes →		then after a further 6 hours 6.25 microgram/kg over 10 minutes	then after a further 6 hours 125–250 microgram over 10 minutes

Oral loading dose

Age	Pre-term newborn infant <1.5kg	Pre-term newborn infant 1.5–2.5kg	Newborn infant to 2 years	2 to 5 years	5 to 10 years	*>10 years
Dose	12.5 microgram/kg	15 microgram/kg	22.5 microgram/kg	17.5 microgram/kg	12.5 microgram/kg (max 375 microgram)	375–750 microgram
	then after 6 hours 6.25 microgram/kg	then after 6 hours 7.5 microgram/kg	then after 6 hours 11.25 microgram/kg	then after 6 hours 8.75 microgram/kg	then after 6 hours 6.25 microgram/kg (max 187.5 microgram)	then after 6 hours 187.5–375 microgram
	then after a further 6 hours 6.25 microgram/kg	then after a further 6 hours 7.5 microgram/kg	then after a further 6 hours 11.25 microgram/kg	then after a further 6 hours 8.75 microgram/kg	then after a further 6 hours 6.25 microgram/kg (max 187.5 microgram)	then after a further 6 hours 187.5–375 microgram

* >10 years use doses at the lower end of the range in early adolescence and/or in underweight children.

Maintenance dose: IV or oral

Age	Pre-term newborn infant <1.5kg	Pre-term newborn infant 1.5–2.5kg	Newborn infant to 2 years	2 to 5 years	5 to 10 years	*>10 years	Frequency (times daily)	Notes
Dose	2.5 microgram/kg	3 microgram/kg	←―5 microgram/kg―→		3 microgram/kg (max 125 microgram)	–	2	The total daily dose may be given once a day.
	–	–	–		–	125–750 microgram	1	

When changing from the IV to the oral route the dose may need to be increased by 20% (liquid) or 30% (tablets) to maintain the same blood levels.

 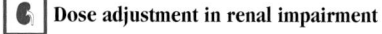 **Dose adjustment in renal impairment**

Grade	Serum creatinine micromol/L (approx)	Creatinine clearance mL/min/1.73m²	Dosage (loading and maintenance)
Mild	150–300	20–50	reduce dose by 50%
Moderate	300–700	10–20	reduce dose by 50%

NOTES

■ **Administration: oral:** do not crush tablets; there is a liquid formulation available (which must not be diluted). **IV:** each dose should be given by slow IV bolus over 10 minutes. The injection may be given undiluted if given slowly over 10 minutes or diluted with a four-fold or greater volume of glucose 5% or NaCl 0.9%. Dilution should be carried out immediately before use and any unused solution discarded.

■ The oral bioavailability of the liquid (80%) and tablets (70%) differs. **When changing from the IV to the oral route the dose may need to be increased by 20% (liquid) or 30% (tablets) to maintain the same blood levels**.

■ Contra-indicated in complete heart block, hypertrophic cardiomyopathy, hypersensitivity to digitalis glycosides and supraventricular arrhythmias associated with an accessory pathway, as in the Wolff-Parkinson-White syndrome.

■ Use with caution in hypokalaemia, hypomagnesaemia, hypercalcaemia, hypertensive heart failure, acute myocardial infarction, direct DC conversion, bradycardia and in combination with quinidine, amiodarone, flecainide, propafenone, spironolactone, tetracycline, erythromycin, verapamil, diltiazem, corticosteroids, diuretics, amphotericin.

■ Therapeutic plasma concentration range is 0.8–2 microgram/L (1-2.6nanomol/L). Levels should be measured in a plasma sample taken at least 6 hours after an oral or IV dose. Approximate time to steady state is 5-10 days.

■ 🔲 Digoxin is licensed for use in all ages with the exception of the 100 microgram in 1mL injection which is available as a 'special' and as such is unlicensed.

124 Dihydrocodeine tartrate

■ **Tablets:** 30mg.
■ **Oral liquid:** 10mg in 5mL.

■ **Injection:** 50mg in 1mL. (controlled drug).

DOSAGE

Route	Age			Frequency (times daily)	Notes
	1 month–2 years	2–12 years	12–18 years		
Oral/IM/ deep SC	≥1 year 500 microgram/kg	≤4 years 500 microgram/kg ≥4 years 500 microgram/kg–1mg/kg	30mg (up to 50mg has been given IM/deep SC)	4–6 hourly 4–6 hourly	Repeated doses increase the risk of respiratory depression. Avoid IM injections if possible. Use SC/IM cannula placed while under GA or topical LA. Dihydrocodeine can cause severe constipation so prophylactic laxatives should always be prescribed.

NOTES

■ Avoid in respiratory depression, cystic fibrosis, head injury or raised intra-cranial pressure.

■ IV administration is not recommended due to increased risk of respiratory depression.

■ Naloxone may be required as an antidote in cases of overdosage.

■ Avoid or reduce dose in moderate to severe renal impairment.

■ Avoid or reduce dose in liver disease; may precipitate coma

■ Licensed for use ≥4 years of age.

■ **Injection:** 12.5mg in 1mL; 20mL vial, 20mL ampoule. 50mg in 1mL; 5mL ampoule.

DOSAGE

Route	Age				Frequency	Notes
	birth–1 month	1 month–2 years	2–12 years	12–18 years		
IV infusion	←	2–10 microgram/kg/minute		→	continuous	Dose can be increased up to a maximum of 15microgram/kg/minute in newborn infants and 40microgram/kg/minute in older children and adults, if necessary.

NOTES

■ **Administration:** solutions must be diluted before use to a maximum concentration of 5mg in 1mL. Direct IV push is not recommended. Must be administered by IV infusion only using an infusion pump to control the flow rate. Diluted solutions should be used within 24 hours. Solution may exhibit pink discoloration without loss of potency for up to 24 hours at room temperature. Compatible with glucose 5% and NaCl 0.9%. Incompatible with alkaline solutions e.g. sodium bicarbonate. Store below 25°C; protect from light.

■ Contra-indicated in idiopathic hypertrophic subaortic stenosis, obstruction to left ventricular filling or emptying, hypovolaemia, cardiac arrhythmias, low cardiac filling pressure.

■ Use with caution in ventricular ectopics, atrial flutter or fibrillation, severe hypotension.

- **Capsules:** 100mg.
- **Oral liquid:** 12.5mg in 5mL, 50mg in 5mL.

- **Enema:** 90mg & glycerol 3.78g in 5mL – Fletcher's enemette®.
- **Enema:** 120mg in 10g – Norgalax Micro-enema®.

DOSAGE

Route	Age			Frequency	Notes
	1 month–2 years	2–12 years	12–18 years	(times daily)	
Oral	>6 months 2.5mg/kg	2.5mg/kg	100mg	3	
Rectal (Fletcher's enemette®)	–	≥3 years one enema	one enema	single dose	As required.
Rectal (Norgalax Micro-enema®)	–	–	one enema	single dose	

NOTES

- **Administration: rectal:** for rectal administration of enema, remove protective cap, insert nozzle into rectum and squeeze gently until tube is empty.

- Onset of action following oral administration is 1-2 days and following rectal administration is within 20 minutes.

- Capsules, 50mg in 5mL oral liquid and the Norgalax Micro-enema® are licensed for use in adults only. The Fletcher's enemette® is licensed for use ≥3 years of age. The 12.5mg in 5mL oral liquid is licensed for use in infants >6 months of age and in children.

■ **Tablets:** 10mg.
■ **Suspension:** 5mg in 5mL.

■ **Suppositories:** 30mg.

DOSAGE

Indication	Route	Age			Frequency (times daily)	Notes
		1 month–2 years	2–12 years	12–18 years		
Gastro-oesophageal reflux, gastric stasis	Oral	←200–400 microgram/kg→		10–20mg	3-4	Not often used <2 years; little data but extrapyramidal effects can occur. Give before food and at night.
Radiotherapy/ chemotherapy induced nausea and vomiting.	Oral	←200–400 microgram/kg→		10–20mg	single dose	Give every 4-8 hours. Not often used <2 years; little data but extrapyramidal effects can occur.
	Rectal	–	15–30mg	30–60mg	single dose	Single dose approximately 1mg/kg. Can repeat doses as below: <25kg repeat up to twice. 25-35kg repeat up to 3 times. >35kg repeat up to 4 times.

NOTES
■ **Administration: rectal:** suppositories may be divided.

■ Only licensed in children for the management of nausea and vomiting following radiotherapy or chemotherapy.

Dopamine hydrochloride

■ **Injection:** 40mg in 1mL; 5mL, 10mL vials & 5mL ampoules. For dilution and use as an IV infusion.
■ **Injection:** 160mg in 1mL; 5mL ampoule. For dilution and use as an IV infusion.

■ **Infusion:** 400mg in 250mL glucose 5%.
■ **Infusion:** 800mg in 250ml glucose 5%.

DOSAGE

Route	Age				Frequency	Notes
	birth–1 month	1 month–2 years	2–12 years	12–18 years		
IV infusion	←	1–5 microgram/kg/minute		→	continuous	Low dose for renal effect. See monograph in *Medicines for Children* as some debate over its use.

DOSAGE continued

Route	Age				Frequency	Notes
	birth–1 month	1 month–2 years	2–12 years	12–18 years		
IV infusion	Start at 3 microgram/kg/minute increasing as clinically indicated to a maximum of 20 microgram/kg/minute	← 5–20 microgram/kg/minute →			continuous	Direct inotropic effect but vasoconstriction may occur at higher doses.

NOTES

■ **Administration: IV:** administer with an infusion pump. It is preferable to dilute dopamine with NaCl 0.9% or glucose 5% before administration, although if fluid restricted, it can be administered undiluted via a syringe pump. Infuse via a central line. Dopamine cannot be mixed with sodium bicarbonate and other strongly alkaline solutions. Dopamine and dobutamine can be mixed together in glucose 5% or NaCl 0.9%. Sodium content: 0.526 mmol per 5mL. pH: 2.5–5.5. Do not use if discoloured.

■ Contra-indicated in patients with phaeochromocytoma, hyperthyroidism, uncorrected arterial or ventricular tachyarrhythmias or ventricular fibrillation.

■ Cyclopropane and halogenated hydrocarbon anaesthetics should be avoided due to arrhythmogenic potential.

■ Use with caution in hypovolaemia, myocardial infarction and in combination with phenytoin or alpha and beta-blockers.

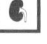

■ **Tablets:** 2.5mg, 5mg, 10mg, 20mg.

DOSAGE

Route	Age				Frequency (times daily)	Notes
	birth–1 month	1 month–2 years	2–12 years	12–18 years		
Oral	40 microgram/kg	← 100 microgram/kg →		2.5mg	1	Initial dose. In neonates it may be necessary to give the total dose in divided doses due to variability in duration of action e.g. 5-10 microgram/kg/**dose** given 1-3 times daily.
	300–500 microgram/kg	← 300 –500 microgram/kg → (maximum 1mg/kg)		10–20mg (maximum 40mg)	1	Maintenance dose. Gradually increase dose according to response.

NOTES

■ See captopril monograph for further information.

■ **Administration: oral:** tablets can be dispersed in water prior to administration.

renal artery stenosis or outflow tract obstruction. Patients with renal impairment may respond to smaller or less frequent dosage. (Titrate dose to response). Removed by dialysis, give 25% of dose after haemodialysis.

■ Enalapril has been substituted for captopril on a basis of 1mg enalapril for every 7.5mg captopril.

■ **Injection:** 100mg (10,000 units) in 1mL; 20mg, 40mg, 60mg, 80mg and 100mg prefilled syringes

■ **Injection:** 150mg (15,000 units) in 1mL; 120mg and 150mg prefilled syringes.

DOSAGE

Indication	Route	Age			Frequency	Notes
		1 month–2 years	2–12 years	12–18 years	(times daily)	
Prophylaxis	SC	<2 months 750 microgram/kg ←— 500 microgram/kg —→ (maximum dose 40mg) ≥2 months 500 microgram/kg			2 2	
Treatment	SC	<2 months 1.5 mg/kg ←— 1mg/kg —→ ≥2 months 1mg/kg			2 2	

Experience is very limited in children.

NOTES

■ In renal impairment no adjustment of the prophylaxis dose is required but patients with severe renal impairment should be closely monitored when receiving treatment doses.

■ In the absence of clinical studies involving hepatic impairment caution should be exercised.

■ As different low molecular weight heparins may not be equivalent, alternative products should not be substituted during a course of treatment.

Ergocalciferol (calciferol, vitamin D₂)

■ **Tablets:** 250 micrograms (10,000 units).

■ **Oral liquid:** several strengths available – manufactured 'specials'.

DOSAGE

Route	Age			Frequency (times daily)	Notes
	1 month–2 years	2–12 years	12–18 years		
Oral	≤ 6 months 3,000 units ≥ 6 months 6,000 units	6,000 units	10,000 units	1 1	

NOTES

- All patients receiving pharmacological doses of vitamin D should have their plasma calcium concentration checked regularly and when nausea and vomiting are present.

- 🔲 Ergocalciferol 250 microgram tablets are licensed for use in children and adults for simple vitamin D deficiency, vitamin D deficiency caused by intestinal malabsorption or chronic liver disease, hypocalcaemia of hypoparathyroidism. Oral liquids are 'specials' and as such are unlicensed.

- Several strengths of oral liquid are available from various hospital manufacturing units.

Erythromycin

- **Suspension:** 125mg in 5mL, 250mg in 5mL, 500mg in 5mL.
- **Tablets:** 250mg, 500mg.
- **Capsules:** 250mg.
- **Topical Solution:** 2% in an alcoholic basis.
- **Topical Gel:** 2%, 4% in an alcoholic basis.
- **Injection:** 1g vial.

DOSAGE

Newborn infant

Route	Age	Frequency (times daily)	Notes
	birth to 1 month		
	12.5mg/kg	4	

Child

Indication	Route	Age			Frequency (times daily)	Notes
		1 month–2 years	2–12 years	12–18 years		
Infection	Oral	125mg	2-8 years 250mg 9-12 years 500mg	500mg	4 4	Doses can be doubled in severe infections. Maximum singe dose 1g.
	IV	←	12.5mg/kg	→	4	
	Topical		–	directly to affected area	2	Apply after washing to the affected area.
Cystic fibrosis patients	Oral		DOSE BY WEIGHT ← 25mg/kg →		2	Treatment of asymptomatic S. aureus isolates or minor exacerbations. Total daily dose can be given in four divided doses.
		250mg	DOSE BY AGE 2-8 years 500mg 8-12 years 1g	1g	2 2	

Child continued

Indication	Route	Age			Frequency	Notes
		1 month–2 years	2–12 years	12–18 years	(times daily)	
Pneumococcal prophylaxis	Oral	125mg	2-8 years 250mg 9-12 years 500mg	500mg	2 2	Used in penicillin allergic patients.
Gastric stasis	Oral/IV	←	3mg/kg	→	4	

NOTES

■ **Administration: oral:** total daily dose may be given in 2 divided doses, but gastrointestinal side effects can occur. **IV:** the addition of 20mL Water for Injections to the 1g vial will give a total volume of 22mL; 20mL of this solution contains 1g erythromycin (i.e. 50mg in 1mL). Dilute 10 times with NaCl 0.9% or neutralised glucose 5% (prepare by adding 5mL of sterile 8.4% w/v sodium bicarbonate to one litre glucose 5% infusion). Infuse over 60 minutes. Total daily dose may be continuously infused over 24 hours at a concentration of 1mg in 1mL (maximum 5mg in 1mL).

■ Increased risk of cardiotoxicity with terfenadine or astemizole.

■ Increased serum concentrations of carbamazepine, digoxin, warfarin, phenytoin, theophylline, ciclosporin, disopyramide, midazolam and alfentanil.

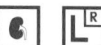

■ **Tablets:** 100mg, 400mg.

■ **Oral liquid:** may be extemporaneously prepared.

DOSAGE

Route	Age			Frequency (times daily)	Notes
	1 month–2 years	2–12 years	12–18 years		
Oral	←	15mg/kg	→	1	The dose given is that used in the standard 6 month regimen of tuberculosis treatment where once daily dosing is used. Maximum dose 1.5g/**day**.

Treatment should always be given in collaboration with a specialist experienced in tuberculosis therapy.

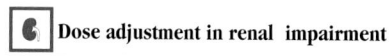 **Dose adjustment in renal impairment**

Creatinine clearance (mL/min/1.73m²)	Dosage
10–50	50% of normal dose
<10	25% of normal dose

Ethambutol is only slightly dialyzable, (5–20%).

NOTES

■ Patients should undergo full ophthalmic examination before starting treatment, including visual acuity, colour vision, perimetry and ophthalmoscopy.

■ Patients who cannot understand warnings about visual side effects should, if possible, be given an alternative drug.

■ Ethambutol should be used with caution in children until they are at least 5 years old and capable of reporting symptomatic visual changes accurately.

■ Ethambutol is licensed for use in adults and children except for the oral liquid, which since it must be extemporaneously prepared, is an unlicensed preparation.

Flucloxacillin

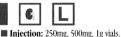

■ **Capsules:** 250mg, 500mg.
■ **Syrup:** 125mg in 5mL, 250mg in 5mL.

■ **Injection:** 250mg, 500mg, 1g vials.

DOSAGE

Newborn infant (birth to 1 month)

Route	Age	Dosage	Frequency (times daily)	Notes
IV/oral	<7 days	25–50mg/kg	2	Dose may be increased to 100mg/kg/dose IV in severe infection (meningitis, cerebral abscess, staphylococcal osteitis). Oral route only recommended for minor infection.
	7–21 days	25–50mg/kg	3	
	>21 days	25–50mg/kg	4	

Child

Route	Age			Frequency (times daily)	Notes
	1 month-2 years	2-12 years	12-18 years		
IV/IM	←	12.5mg-25mg/kg	→	4	Maximum single dose 1g. For severe infection, doses may be doubled up to a maximum single dose of 2g.
Oral	≤1 year 62.5mg >1 year 125mg	≤5 years 125mg >5 years 250mg	250mg	4 4	Doses may be doubled in severe infection.
Oral for cystic fibrosis patients	← 16-33mg/kg	→	1g	4	Continuous anti-staphylococcal therapy. To aid compliance usually given in two divided doses but ideally given four times daily.
	←	12.5-25mg/kg	→	4	Treatment of asymptomatic *S. aureus* isolates or minor exacerbations. Maximum single dose of 1g. Daily dose can be given in three divided doses if necessary.

NOTES

■ **Administration: oral:** give at least 30 minutes before food. The powder can be shaken out of the capsule for patients allergic to colours and preservatives. The syrup can be diluted with Syrup BP. **IM & IV:** on reconstitution 250mg displaces 0.2mL. IM injection - add 1.3mL Water for Injections to 250mg vial to give 250mg in 1.5mL and 1.6mL to 500mg vial to give 500mg in 2mL. IV bolus – dilute reconstituted dose to 5-10mL with Water for Injections and give over 3-5 minutes. Do not mix with aminoglycosides; do not administer through the same line without adequate flushing in-between.

■ If creatinine clearance is <10mL/min/1.73m², increase the dosage interval.

■ Contra-indicated in penicillin hypersensitivity.

■ Injection: each 1g of powder contains 2.26mmol of sodium.

Fluconazole

■ **Capsules:** 50mg, 150mg, 200mg.
■ **Oral suspension:** 50mg in 5mL, 200mg in 5mL.
■ **IV infusion:** 2mg in 1mL in NaCl 0.9% (25mL, 100mL).

DOSAGE

Newborn infant (birth to 1 month)

Route	Age	Dose	Frequency	Notes
Oral/IV	<14 days	6–12mg/kg	every 72 hours	Systemic candidiasis and cryptococcal infection. Dose can be reduced to 3mg/kg with the same dosage intervals to treat mucosal candidiasis. Well absorbed orally when gastrointestinal function is adequate.
	14–28 days	6–12mg/kg	every 48 hours	
	>28 days	6–12mg/kg	every 24 hours	

Child

Route	Age			Frequency	Notes
	1 month–2 years	2–12 years	12–18 years	(times daily)	
Oral/IV	→	6mg/kg	←	single dose	Loading dose.
	→	then 3mg/kg	←	1	Mucosal candidiasis for 7–14 days.
	→	6–12mg/kg	←	1	Systemic candidiasis and cryptococcal infection; dose depends on severity. Maximum dose 400mg.
	→	3–12mg/kg	←	1	Prevention of fungal infection in immunocompromised patients; dose depends on extent and duration of neutropenia. Maximum dose 400mg.

Dose adjustment in renal impairment

Give normal dose on day 1 to achieve therapeutic levels then:

Creatinine clearance (mL/min/1.73m²)	Dosage
10–50	Reduce dose by 50% or give normal dose every 48 hours
<10	Reduce dose to one third of the normal dose or give normal dose every 72 hours

NOTES

■ **Administration: IV:** give as an IV infusion over 10-30 minutes. Compatible with Ringers solution, Hartmann's solution, sodium bicarbonate 4.2%, NaCl 0.9% or glucose solutions.

Fluquincodrtisone acetate

■ **Tablets:** 100 microgram
■ **Capsules:** 1mg, 5mg; available as 'specials'.
■ **Oral liquid:** may be extemporaneously prepared.

DOSAGE

Indication	Route	Age				Frequency (times daily)	Notes
		birth– 1 month	1 month– 2 years	2-12 years	12-18 years		
Adrenal insufficiency	Oral	←	50-200 microgram		→	1	**Replacement therapy** Adjust according to response.
Sweat test	Oral	←	$3mg/m^2$		→	1	Two doses given on consecutive days prior to sweat test.

NOTES

■ L▣ Tablets are licensed for replacement therapy in all ages; not for sweat test.

The capsules are available as 'specials' from Mandeville Medicines and are therefore unlicensed.

Flumazenil

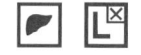

■ **Injection:** 500 microgram in 5mL.

DOSAGE

Route	Age				Frequency	Notes
	birth– 1 month	1 month– 2 years	2–12 years	12–18 years		
IV bolus over 15 seconds	10 microgram/kg	← 10 microgram/kg → (maximum of 200 microgram dose)		200 microgram dose	single dose	Initial dose. If the desired effect is not achieved - repeat at 1 minute intervals to a **maximum total dose** of 40 microgram/kg (2mg dose).
IV infusion	← 2–10 microgram/kg/hour →			100–400 microgram/hour	continuous	This should be individually adjusted to achieve the desired level of arousal.

There is limited experience of the use of flumazenil in children.

NOTES

■ **Administration: IV:** initial dose is administered over 15 seconds. This may be repeated after 1 minute if the desired level of consciousness is not obtained. May be diluted with glucose 5% or NaCl 0.9%. Infusion may be necessary if drowsiness returns after single doses.

■ Careful titration of the dose is necessary in hepatic failure. Initial dose is the same but subsequent doses may be reduced in size and frequency.

Fluticasone propionate

■ **Aerosol inhaler:** 25 microgram per actuation.
■ **CFC-free inhaler:** 50, 125, 250 microgram per actuation.
■ **Nebules:** 500 microgram in 2mL; 2mg in 2mL.

■ **Breath-actuated inhaler:** 50, 100, 250, 500 microgram per actuation or per blister.
■ **Aqueous nasal spray:** 50 microgram per metered spray.

DOSAGE

Route	Age		Frequency	Notes
	2–12 years	12–18 years	(times daily)	
Inhaled	<u>≤4 years</u> 50–100 microgram	<u>12–16 years</u> 50–200 microgram	2	<u>Asthma:</u> the starting dose should be appropriate to the severity of the disease. The dosage should be adjusted until control is achieved and then reduced to the minimum effective dose according to individual response.
	≥4 years 50–200 microgram	≥16 years 100 microgram - 1mg	2	

Route	Age		Frequency (times daily)	Notes
	2–12 years	12–18 years		
Nebulised	1mg	<u>12–16 years</u> 1mg	2	<u>Asthma</u>: acute exacerbation of asthma.
	-	<u>≥16 years</u> 500 microgram-2mg	2	<u>Asthma</u>: prophylactic management of chronic severe asthma in patients requiring high dose inhaled or oral corticosteroid therapy.
Intra-nasal	<u>≥4 years</u> 50 micrograms (1spray) into each nostril	100 micrograms (2 sprays) into each nostril	1	<u>Allergic rhinitis:</u> Twice daily dosing may be required.

NOTES

■ **Administration: Inhaler:** fluticasone aerosol inhaler can be used via a large volume spacer (Volumatic®, Babyhaler®) and mask for infants and young children. Administration of doses above 500 micrograms twice daily from the Evohaler® should also be administered via a large volume spacer.
Nebulised: via a jet nebuliser. Preferably with a mouthpiece to avoid atrophic changes to facial skin which may occur with prolonged use of a facemask. If a facemask is used the exposed skin should be protected with a barrier cream or the face should be thoroughly washed after treatment.

■ Rinse mouth well after use of inhalers to reduce hoarseness and throat irritation.

■ 🅛🅡 Preparations for inhalation containing ≤100 microgram/actuation are licensed for use ≥4 years of age; those containing ≥125 microgram/actuation are not licensed for use in children. Nebules are licensed for use ≥16 years of age.

■ **Tablets:** 400 microgram, 5mg.

■ **Syrup:** 2.5mg in 5mL; 400 microgram in 5mL.

DOSAGE

Newborn infant: preterm babies fed heat-treated human milk may benefit from a 500 microgram supplement once a week unless a suitable breast milk fortifier is used. Supplementation has no impact on the risk of anaemia developing in other term or preterm breast or formula fed babies.

Indication	Route	Age				Frequency (times daily)	Notes
		birth– 1 month	1 month– 2 years	2–12 years	12–18 years		
Supplementation – in folate deficiency in infants and children; co-factor in metabolic disorders e.g. homocystinuria	Oral	← 250 microgram/kg →			5–10mg	1	For 6 months if a correctable cause; for life if an uncorrectable cause.

L

DOSAGE continued

Indication	Route	Age				Frequency (times daily)	Notes
		birth–1 month	1 month–2 years	2–12 years	12–18 years		
Treatment of megaloblastic anaemia due to folate deficiency	Oral	1mg	**DOSE BY WEIGHT** <u><1 year</u> 500 microgram/kg **DOSE BY AGE** <u>1–2 years</u> 5mg	← 5mg →		1 1	For up to 4 months. For maintenance therapy the treatment doses may be given at daily to weekly intervals.
Haemolytic anaemia	Oral	-	← 2.5–5mg →		10mg	1	Seek haematologist's advice.

NOTES
- Before treating megaloblastic anaemia with folic acid, vitamin B12 deficiency must be excluded, as neuropathy may be precipitated.

■ **Tablets:** 20mg, 40mg, 500mg.
■ **Oral solution:** 1mg in 1mL, 20mg in 5mL, 40mg in 5mL, 50mg in 5mL.
■ **Injection:** 20mg in 2mL, 50mg in 5mL, 250mg in 25mL.

DOSAGE

Route	Age				Frequency (times daily)	Notes
	birth–1 month	1 month–2 years	2–12 years	12–18 years		
Oral	500 microgram/kg – 1mg/kg	–	–	–	2	Larger doses sometimes necessary but do not exceed maximum single dose of 6mg/kg/dose.
	–	← 1–2mg/kg →		20–40mg	2–3	Repeat as necessary.
IV bolus	← 500 microgram/kg – 1mg/kg →			20–40mg	single dose	Single doses up to 4mg/kg have been used. Dose can be repeated every 8 hours.
IV infusion	–	100 microgram/kg/hour – ← 2mg/kg/hour →		not exceeding 4mg/minute	continuous	IV infusion for paediatric post operative cardiac patients – an initial dose of 100 microgram/kg/hour is suggested, doubling the dose every 2 hours until urine output exceeds 1mL/kg/hour, up to a maximum dose of 2mg/kg/hour.

NOTES

■ **Administration: IV:** may be given as a bolus over at least 2 minutes or as an infusion.

■ Higher doses than normal may be required in patients with renal failure and hepatic insufficiency.

■ Furosemide is incompatible with glucose solutions but may be mixed with NaCl 0.9%.

Gabapentin

■ **Capsules:** 100mg, 300mg, 400mg

■ **Tablets:** 600mg, 800mg.

DOSAGE

Route	Age				Frequency (times daily)	Notes
	birth–1 month	1 month–2 years	2–12 years	12–18 years		
Oral	–	–	10mg/kg	300mg	see notes	<u>Starting dose.</u> Give once daily on day 1, twice daily on day 2 and three times daily on day 3 increasing to maintenance. Note: some children may not tolerate daily increments and up to weekly increases may be more appropriate.
	–	–	10–20mg/kg	300–800mg	3	<u>Target maintenance dose.</u> May be effective given twice daily. Doses up to 70mg/kg/**day** may

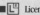

Dose adjustment for renal impairment

Creatinine clearance (mL/minute/1.73m²)	Frequency of maintenance dose
30-60	twice a day
15-30	once daily
<15	once daily on alternate days

Haemodialysis: 8-12mg/kg loading dose then 6-8mg/kg after each 4 hour dialysis period.

NOTES
- **Administration:** capsules can be opened but contents are very bitter and difficult to mask even with blackcurrant or cola drinks. Concomitant antacids reduce absorption. Absorption is unaffected by food.

- Licensed for use > 6 years of age.

■ **Capsules:** 250mg, 500mg.
■ **Oral suspension:** may be extemporaneously prepared.

■ **Injection:** 500mg vial for reconstitution and use as an infusion.

DOSAGE

Newborn infant (birth to 1 month)

Route	Age		Frequency (times daily)	Notes
	Up to 7 days	Over 7 days		
IV	← 5mg/kg →		2	Reduce frequency in renal impairment and very low birth weight infants.

Child

Route	Age			Frequency (times daily)	Notes
	1 month-2 years	2-12 years	12-18 years		
Oral	← 20-40mg/kg →		1g	3	Give with food to maximise absorption. Unlicensed in children <12 years.
IV	← 5mg/kg →			2	Induction regime for 14–21 days if treatment of CMV or 7 to14 days if used in prevention of CMV in at risk patients.
	← 5mg/kg →			1	Maintenance For 7 days a week
	← 6mg/kg →			1	For 5 days a week

Dose adjustment in renal impairment
IV induction

Creatinine clearance (mL/min/1.73m²)	Dose	Frequency (times daily)
50–80	2.5mg/kg	2
10–50	2.5mg/kg	1
<10	1.25mg/kg	1

Haemodialysis patients should be given 1.25mg/kg every 24 hours. Doses should be given shortly after dialysis session as ganciclovir is removed by dialysis.

Maintenance
Manufacturer has no recommendation but the following have been used:
IV maintenance (all ages)

Creatinine clearance (mL/min/1.73m²)	Dose	Frequency (times daily)
50–70	2.5mg/kg	2
25–49	2.5mg/kg	1
10–24	1.25mg/kg	1

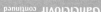

Oral maintenance (12–18 years)

Creatinine clearance (mL/min/1.73m²)	Dose	Frequency
50–69	1.5g	once daily
25–49	1g	once daily
10–24	500mg	once daily
<10	500mg	3 times weekly

NOTES

■ **Administration: IV:** reconstitute each vial with 10mL Water for Injections to give 50mg in 1mL. Displacement value is negligible. Infuse over 1 hour at a concentration of no more than 10mg in 1mL. Compatible with NaCl 0.9%, glucose 5%, compound sodium lactate.

■ Caution is advised when handling ganciclovir as the reconstituted solution is irritant (pH = 11). Ganciclovir is also potentially carcinogenic and teratogenic. Gloves and eye protection are recommended.

■ Injection contains 2mmol sodium in each 500mg vial.

■ Avoid in pregnancy.

■ Do not breast feed until 72 hours after the last dose of ganciclovir.

■ Injection is unlicensed for use in neonates; licensed for use in the treatment of cytomegalovirus infections; treatment of other potentially susceptible viral infections is unlicensed. Capsules are unlicensed for use < 12 years of age. Oral suspension may be extemporaneously prepared and as such is unlicensed.

- **Tablets:** alginic acid 500mg, anhydrous aluminium hydroxide 100mg, magnesium trisilicate 25mg, sodium bicarbonate 170mg. Lemon or peppermint flavour.
- **Liquid:** sodium alginate 250mg, sodium bicarbonate 133.5mg, calcium carbonate 80mg in 5mL. Peppermint or aniseed flavour.
- **Infant sachets:** oral powder containing: sodium alginate 225mg, anhydrous aluminium hydroxide 112.5g with colloidal silica and mannitol, magnesium alginate 87.5mg per dose (half dual sachet).
- **Suspension:** sodium alginate 500mg, potassium bicarbonate 100mg in 5mL; peppermint or aniseed flavour - Gaviscon® Advance

DOSAGE

Route	Age				Frequency	Notes
	birth– 1 month	1 month– 2 years	2–12 years	12–18 years		
Oral	≤4.5 kg ← 1 dose (½ dual sachet) → ≥4.5 kg ← 2 doses (1 dual sachet) →		1 tablet or 5–10mL liquid	1-2 tablets or 10-20mL liquid	single dose	Give infant sachets with/after feeds. to a maximum of 6 times per day. >2 years give liquid or oral tablets after meals and at bedtime.
Oral	-	-	-	5–10mL	single dose	≥12 years of age Gaviscon® Advance after meals and at bedtime.

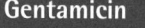

NOTES

■ **Administration: tablets:** may be crushed, chewed or mixed with food or drink. **Infant sachets:** mix with milk feed. In breast-fed infants, add 5mL boiled, cooled water to powder, mix to a smooth paste, add 2 X 5mL spoonfuls of water and give from a spoon during or after a feed.

■ Infants less than 2 years should only receive sachets since they contain less sodium than other preparations.

■ Liquid and tablets are licensed for use ≥2 years (2 - 6 years use only on medical advice). Infant sachets are licensed for infants and young children (<1 year of age only under medical supervision).

■ Do not use Gaviscon Infant with thickening agents or infant milk preparations containing a thickening agent as it could lead to over thickening of the stomach contents.

Gentamicin

Many dosage regimens exist for aminoglycosides depending on target concentrations aimed for and patient groups treated. The dosage regimens shown here are generally accepted initial doses and adjustments should be made in light of serum concentration measurement.

■ **Injection:** 10mg in 1mL; 2mL vial. 40mg in 1mL; 1mL amp, 2mL amp or vial, 6mL vial.

■ **Intrathecal Injection:** 5mg in 1mL.
■ **Ear Drops:** 0.3% w/v.

DOSAGE
Newborn infant (birth - 1 month)
Extended dosing regimen

Route	Postconceptional age	Dose	Frequency (times daily)	Notes
IV	<32 weeks	4-5mg/kg	36 hourly	Plasma samples usually taken around the third dose aiming for a 1 hour post dose (peak) of 5-10mg/L and a pre dose (trough) level of <2mg/L If there is no change in the dosage regimen or renal function repeat levels every 3-4 days.
	>32 weeks	4-5mg/kg	24 hourly	

Postconceptional age = gestational age plus postnatal age.
Neonates presenting with patent ductus arteriosus (PDA), prolonged hypoxia or treated with indometacin may have impaired elimination of gentamicin due to reduced glomerular filtration rate (GFR) and increase in dosage interval may be necessary.

Intrathecal dose

Newborn infant (birth – 1 month)

Route	Age	Dose	Frequency	Notes
Intrathecal	birth to 1 month	1–2mg	every 24 to 48 hours	Only preservative free intrathecal preparation should be used. Aim for CSF level of 5–10mg/L

Child

Divided daily dose regimen

Route	Age			Frequency (times daily)	Notes
	1 month–2 years	2–12 years	12–18 years		
IV/IM	← 2.5mg/kg →		1–2mg/kg	3	Plasma samples usually taken around the third or fourth dose aiming for a pre dose (trough) level of <2mg/L and a 1 hour post dose (peak) 5–10mg/L
Intrathecal or intra-ventricular	← 1mg →			1	Assess MIC of infecting organism and adjust dose to ensure adequate levels are maintained. May be increased if necessary to 5mg. CSF level should not exceed 10mg/L. Accompanied by systemic therapy.

GENTAMICIN continued

Child: Divided daily dose regimen

Route	Age			Frequency (times daily)	Notes
	1 month–2 years	2–12 years	12–18 years		
Nebulised	40mg	<8 years 80mg	160mg	2	Use preservative-free (phenol-free) formulations. Administer after physiotherapy and bronchodilators.
		>8 years 160mg		2	
IV for cystic fibrosis patients	←	3mg/kg	→	3	Starting dose. Monitor blood levels after the third dose. Aim for a trough of <1mg/L and 1 hour post dose (peak) of 8–12mg/L

Single daily dose regimen

Route	Age			Frequency (times daily)	Notes
	1 month–2 years	2–12 years	12–18 years		
IV	←	7mg/kg	→	1	Plasma samples are usually taken at 18–24 hours after the first dose aiming for a level <1mg/L. If the levels are >1mg/L then the dosing interval is normally increased by 12 hours. 1 hour post dose (peak) levels can be taken with a target range of 16–20mg/L. If there is no change in the dosage regimen or in renal function repeat levels every 3–4 days.

NOTES

- **Administration: IV**: slow IV injection over 3-5 minutes injected neat or diluted in NaCl 0.9% or glucose 5%. IV infusion over 30-60 minutes for high dose 'child – single daily dose regimen' in an appropriate volume of fluid. Compatible with NaCl 0.9% and 0.45%, glucose 5% & 10% and glucose 4%/NaCl 0.18%. In general, gentamicin injection should not be mixed with penicillins, cephalosporins, erythromycin, heparin or sodium bicarbonate. Adequate flushing or administration at separate sites is suggested. **Nebulised:** optimum nebuliser volume is 3mL; make up volume with NaCl 0.9%. May be mixed with colistin; add gentamicin dose to the colistin vial immediately before use and then make up to 3mL with NaCl 0.9%. **Intrathecal:** only the intrathecal preparation should be used. **Ear drops:** 2-3 drops 3-4 times daily and at night; do not use if there is perforation of the ear drum.

- In patients with impaired renal function dosage and/or frequency of administration must be adjusted in response to serum drug concentrations and the extent of renal impairment.

Glucagon

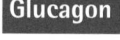

- **Injection:** 1mg vial with Water for Injections in prefilled syringe.

DOSAGE

Indication	Route	Age				Frequency	Notes
		birth–1 month	1 month–2 years	2–12 years	12–18 years	(times daily)	
Severe hypo-glycaemia in the treatment	IM SC IV raid	20 microgram/kg	500 microgram	500 microgram - 1mg (< 25kg: 500 microgram)		single dose	Should be effective within 15 minutes. If not, give IV glucose 5-10%.

Glycopyronium bromide

■ **Tablets:** 1mg, 2mg (both scored) - named patient.

■ **Injection:** 200 microgram in 1mL; 1mL and 3mL ampoule.

■ **Injection:** 500 microgram in 1mL with neostigmine 2.5mg; 1mL ampoule.

DOSAGE

Indication	Route	Age				Frequency	Notes
		birth–1 month	1 month–2 years	2–12 years	12–18 years	(times daily)	
Premedication and intra-operative use	IM/IV	–	← 4-8 microgram/kg →			single dose	Maximum dose 200 micrograms; larger doses may result in profound and prolonged antisialogogue effect.
Antagonism of neostigmine muscarinic effects	IV	–	← 10 microgram/kg →			single dose	With 50 microgram/kg neostigmine using the combined preparation. Used for reversal of residual non-depolarising neuromuscular block.

DOSAGE *continued*

Indication	Route	Age				Frequency (times daily)	Notes
		birth–1 month	1 month–2 years	2–12 years	12–18 years		
Control of upper airway secretions	Oral	–	← 40–100 microgram/kg →			3–4	Note: oral dose is 10 times the parenteral dose.

NOTES

- **Administration: IM:** use undiluted injection 30–60 minutes prior to anaesthetic. **IV:** use undiluted injection at induction. **Oral:** injection can be given orally. Tablets can be dispersed in water.
- Use is contra-indicated in patients with urinary tract obstruction, ileus or pyloric stenosis.

- L.E. Licensed for use in children and adults as pre-medication and for reversal of neuromuscular block as the combined preparation with neostigmine. Tablets are not licensed for use in the UK.
- Tablets can be obtained via IDIS World Medicines.

Tablets: 125mg, 500mg.

Suspension: 125mg in 5mL.

DOSAGE

Route	Age			Frequency (times daily)	Notes
	1 month-2 years	2-12 years	12-18 years		
Oral	← 10mg/kg →		500mg	1	Local resistance may require doses up to 20mg/kg.

NOTES

■ To be taken with or after food.

■ Avoid pregnancy during treatment and for one month after.

■ Griseofulvin tablets are licensed for use in adults and children; the suspension, which is not a licensed product in the UK, may be imported into the UK on a named patient basis via IDIS.

Heparin (standard or unfractionated)

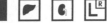

Injection: 1,000 units in 1mL; 1mL, 5mL, 10mL, 20mL ampoules, 5mL vial
5,000 units in 1mL; 1mL, 5mL ampoules, 5ml vial;
25,000 units in 1mL; 0.2mL, 1mL ampoules, 5mL vial.

Subcutaneous injection: 25,000 units in 1mL; 0.2mL, 0.5mL syringes and 0.2mL ampoule.

Flush solutions: 100 units in 1mL; 2mL ampoule.
10 units in 1mL; 5mL ampoule.
There are many preparations of heparin available - see *Medicines for Children* for full details.

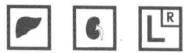

DOSAGE

Indication	Route	Age				Frequency (times daily)	Notes
		birth– 1 month	1 month– 2 years	2–12 years	12–18 years		
Anticoagulant treatment	IV	≤35 weeks postconceptional age: 50 units/kg ≥35 weeks postconceptional age: 75 units/kg	←	75 units/kg	→	single dose	Loading dose.
	IV infusion	25 units/kg/hour	≤1 year as neonate ≥1 year as older child	← 20 units/kg/hour →		continuous	Initial maintenance dose. Adjust subsequent dose to achieve required APTT level.
	SC	–	←	250 units/kg	→	2	
Anticoagulant prophylaxis	SC	–	←	100 units/kg	→	2	Maximum single dose 5,000 units.

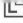

NOTES

■ **Administration:** IV infusion: dilute with glucose 5% or NaCl 0.9%.

■ In severe renal and hepatic impairment the risk of bleeding is increased and dose reduction should be considered.

■ Monitor activated partial thromboplastin time (APTT) and adjust dose to keep within therapeutic range according to local guidelines.

■ Haemorrhage is the major sign of overdose - protamine is the antidote.

■ **Heparin** Calciparine®, Monoparin®, Multiparin®, licensed for use in children (for 'treatment') and adults. Minihep®, Monoparin Calcium® and Pump-Hep® are not recommended for use in children; for adults only. **Heparin flushes:** Heplok®, Hepsal® and Hep-Flush® are not licensed for use in children, Canusal® is licensed for use in children.

■ Heparin flushes have a clear role to maintain patency of arterial catheters. For peripheral venous lines heparin flushes offer no advantage over NaCl 0.9%. Consult local guidelines for individual hospital protocols.

Human albumin solution

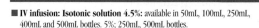

■ **IV infusion: Isotonic solution 4.5%:** available in 50mL, 100mL, 250mL, 400mL and 500mL bottles. 5%; 250mL, 500mL bottles.

■ **IV infusion: concentrated solutions 20-25%:** 20% available in 50mL, 100mL vials/bottles; 25% available in 20mL, 50mL, 100mL bottles.

DOSAGE

For plasma replacement: in hypovolaemic shock 10-20mL/kg of the **isotonic solution** rapidly. Repeat as necessary. In trauma these requirements may increase to 40mL/kg. At this level, replacement with whole blood should be considered.

For diuretic resistant oedema e.g. nephrotic syndrome: 500mg/kg – 1g/kg of the **concentrated solution** over 4 hours with close monitoring with pulse oximetry because of the risk of pulmonary oedema.

NOTES

■ Contra-indicated in severe anaemia and cardiac failure. Extreme caution in babies with congenital heart defects.

■ Large doses may cause pulmonary oedema.

■ Authors (Cochrane Injuries Group Albumin Reviewers) of a review of human albumin administration in critically ill patients, published in the *BMJ* July 1998, concluded that 'there is no evidence that albumin administration reduces mortality in critically ill patients with hypovolaemia burns, or hypoalbuminaemia and a strong suggestion that it may increase mortality. These data suggest that the use of human albumin in critically ill patients should be urgently reviewed'. In the light of this publication and subsequent reaction to it, the information on the use of human albumin contained in this formulary may need to be amended.

Hydralazine

■ **Tablets:** 10mg, 25mg, 50mg.
■ **Tablets (dispersible):** 10mg.

■ **Oral liquid:** may be extemporaneously prepared.
■ **Injection:** 20mg ampoule.

DOSAGE

Route	Age				Frequency	Notes
	birth–1 month	1 month–2 years	2–12 years	12–18 years	(times daily)	
Oral	→	250–500 microgram/kg	←		2–3	Starting dose: increase gradually to a dose not

DOSAGE continued

Route	Age				Frequency (times daily)	Notes
	birth–1 month	1 month–2 years	2–12 years	12–18 years		
Slow IV bolus over 20 minutes	←——— 100–500 microgram/kg ———→			5–10mg	single dose	Can be repeated up to a maximum of 4-6 times daily.
IV infusion	←——— 12.5–50 microgram/kg/hour ———→			3–9mg/hour	continuous	

NOTES

■ **Administration: oral:** the injection can be given orally. **IV:** the contents of the vial should be reconstituted by dissolving in 1mL of Water for Injections. This should then be further diluted with NaCl 0.9% and given by slow IV injection or infusion. Glucose solutions should not be used.

■ Contra-indicated in high output heart failure, porphyria and lupus.

■ Blood dyscrasia and a lupus-like syndrome may occur.

■ The 10mg dispersible tablets are available as a 'special' from Special Products Limited and are therefore unlicensed. The 10mg tablet may be imported via IDIS World Medicines

■ **Tablets:** 10mg, 20mg.
■ **Pellets (lozenges):** 2.5mg.
■ **Oral liquid:** 10mg in 5mL.
■ **Injection:** 100mg in 1mL.
■ **Rectal foam:** 10%w/w.

DOSAGE

Indication	Route	Age				Frequency (times daily)	Notes
		birth – 1 month	1 month – 2 years	2–12 years	12–18 years		
Emergency treatment of severe acute asthma. Anaphylaxis	IV bolus/ IM/intra-osseous	2.5mg/kg then 2mg/kg	← 4mg/kg → (maximum 100mg) then ← 2–4mg/kg →		100–300mg then 100–300mg	single dose then 4	Maintenance dose may be repeated if necessary every 6 hours. May be given by intraosseous route if IV not possible.
Replacement therapy *	Oral	← 4–5mg/m² →				3	Maintenance.
		← 5–6.6mg/m² →				3	Larger replacement dose in congenital adrenal hyperplasia.
Topical treatment of ulcerative colitis, procto-sigmoiditis, granular	Rectal	–	–	–	1 application 125mg	1–2	Daily for 2–3 weeks then once on alternate days.

DOSAGE continued

Indication	Route	Age				Frequency (times daily)	Notes
		birth – 1 month	1 month – 2 years	2–12 years	12–18 years		
Refractory hypotension	IV	2.5mg/kg	-	-	-	4-6	Once stable wean gradually over 2-4 days. Monitor blood glucose and electrolytes.

NOTES

■ **Administration: oral:** take after food in order to minimise gastrointestinal side effects. **IV: IV bolus** - give over 3-5 minutes; **IV infusion** - dilute the prescribed dose in NaCl 0.9% or glucose 5%.

■ Use is contra-indicated in patients with systemic infection, unless specific anti-infective therapy is used.

■ Live vaccines should not be given to patients receiving immunosuppressive doses of steroids.

■ *Replacement therapy doses of hydrocortisone should be increased during acute stress of intercurrent illness with pyrexia, or anaesthesia.

■ **Withdrawal of corticosteroids:** in patients who have received systemic corticosteroids for greater than 3 weeks, withdrawal should not be abrupt. However, abrupt withdrawal is appropriate in some patients treated for up to 3 weeks if it is considered that the disease is unlikely to relapse or that the dose has been such that abrupt withdrawal is unlikely to lead to clinically relevant hypothalamic-pituitary-adrenal axis suppression.

■ The pellets are not licensed for the indications stated. The oral liquid may be imported into the UK or extemporaneously prepared and is therefore unlicensed. Refractory hypotension is not a licensed indication.

L R

■ **Patches:** self-adhesive 2.5cm², 1.5mg; drug released at a rate of 1mg over 72 hours.

■ **Tablets:** 150 micrograms, 300 micrograms.

■ **Injection:** 400 microgram per 1mL, 600 microgram per 1mL; both 1mL ampoules.

DOSAGE

Route	Age			Frequency (times daily)	Notes
	1 month–2 years	2–12 years	12–18 years		
Oral or sublingual	–	10 microgram/kg	300 microgram	4	Can use tablets or the injection orally.
Topical	¼ patch	2–3 years ¼ patch 3–9 years ½ patch 10–12 years 1 patch	1 patch	Once every 72 hours	Apply to the dry, hairless skin behind the ear. Alternate sites each time a new patch is applied. Clean the skin well after patch is taken off to remove any residue. Wash hands after application. Tolerance may develop, so that patches need changing every 48 hours.
SC/IV bolus	← 10 microgram/kg →		400 microgram	4	
SC/IV infusion	← 40–60 microgram/kg/day →			continuous over 24 hours	This is compatible in a syringe with diamorphine.

NOTES

■ **Administration: Patch:** apply to a clean, dry hairless area (e.g. behind ear). Patches may be cut if required, provided that they are cut along their full thickness with scissors and the membrane is not peeled away, the controlled release properties of the patch remain unaltered. Or, the portion of the patch that is not required, can be covered so that it is not in touch with the skin. **Tablet:** can be sucked, chewed or swallowed.

■ Scopoderm TTS® patches are not licensed for the control of drooling but they are licensed for >10 years of age for motion sickness. Transcop® patches are not licensed for use in the UK. Tablets are licensed for ≥3 years of age for motion sickness.

■ Hyoscine is contra-indicated in patients with glaucoma.

UL

■ **Gel:** glucose gel – 10g/23g oral ampoule.

DOSAGE /ADMINISTRATION

For all age groups massage half the contents of an oral ampoule into the buccal cavity. Repeat if there is no clinical response within 10 minutes.

NOTES
■ Do not use in unconscious patients.

■ It may be used in semi-conscious patients in whom the swallowing reflex is present.

Ibuprofen

■ **Tablets:** 200mg, 400mg, 600mg.
■ **Tablets (modified release):** 800mg.
■ **Capsules (modified release):** 300mg.
■ **Injection:** 5mg in 1mL, 2mL ampoules.

■ **Oral liquid:** 100mg in 5mL.
■ **Granules:** 600mg/sachet.
■ **Gel:** 5%.

Indication	Route	Age			Frequency (times daily)	Notes
		1 month– 2 years	2–12 years	12–18 years		
Pyrexia, mild to	Oral	← 5mg/kg →		200–600mg	3–4	Maximum of 20mg/kg/**day** up to 2.4g/**day**.

DOSAGE

Indication	Route	Age			Frequency (times daily)	Notes
		1 month–2 years	2–12 years	12–18 years		
JIA and other rheumatic diseases	Oral	←—	10 mg/kg	—→	3–4	Can be given up to six times daily in systemic JIA only.
Rheumatic and muscular pain	Topical	Not recommended	←— Small amount —→		2–3	

NOTES

■ **Administration: oral**: take with or after food or milk.

■ Avoid in patients with active peptic ulcer disease and in patients who have previously shown hypersensitivty reactions (asthma, rhinitis, urticaria) to aspirin or other NSAIDs.

■ **C** **P** Use with caution in patients with renal impairment, or severe liver impairment.

■ **L** Not licensed for use in children < 7kg or < 6 months of age. Topical preparations, granules and 800mg m/r tablets are not licensed in children. Check individual products for further information.

■ Injection is a 'special' formulated for use IV in closure of patent ductus arteriosus - see *Medicines for Children* for details.

■ **Available as:** 500mg, 2.5g, 3g, 5g, 10g. See *Medicines for Children* for product details.

DOSAGE

Indication	Route	Age				Frequency	Notes
		birth–1 month	1 month–2 years	2–12 years	12–18 years		
ITP	IV infusion	←	800mg/kg – 1g/kg		→	once daily	For 1 – 2 days. Courses should only be repeated only in the presence of symptoms rather than according to platelet count.
Kawasaki Syndrome	IV infusion	–	←	2g/kg →	–	single dose	Give over 12 hours (if rate in the product SPC permits) as soon as possible after onset of disease. Consider second dose if still pyrexial 48 hours later.
Replacement therapy in immuno-deficiency syndrome	IV infusion	–	←	400mg/kg	→	once every 3 weeks	Dose is initially determined by severity and frequency of infections as well as the serum IgG concentration.

For other indications and more detailed information refer to *Medicines for Children*.

Indometacin (indomethacin)

- **Tablets (modified release):** 25mg, 50mg, 75mg.
- **Capsules:** 25mg, 50mg.
- **Capsules (modified release):** 25mg, 75mg, 100mg.
- **Suspension:** 25mg in 5mL.
- **Suppositories:** 100mg.
- **Injection:** 1mg vial.

DOSAGE

Indication	Route	Age				Frequency (times daily)	Notes
		birth– 1 month	1 month– 2 years	2–12 years	12–18 years		
Pain/ inflammation in rheumatic disease	Oral/rectal	–	←————500 microgram/kg - 1mg/kg ————→ (maximum 50mg dose)			2	If modified release, give in 2 divided doses or once only with the evening meal.

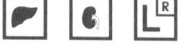

DOSAGE continued

Indication	Route	Age				Frequency (times daily)	Notes
		birth– 1 month	1 month– 2 years	2–12 years	12–18 years		
Nephrogenic diabetes insipidus	Oral	◄—— 500 microgram/kg– 1mg/kg ——►		–	–	2	Amiloride is used in older children.

Newborn infant

Indication: closure of patent ductus arterious (PDA). A course of therapy is defined as three intravenous doses given at 12-24 hour intervals.

Age at first dose	Intravenous dosage (microgram/kg)		
	1st dose	2nd dose	3rd dose
Less than 48 hours	200	100	100
2–7 days	200	200	200
over 7 days	200	250	250

If anuria or marked oliguria (urinary output of 0.6 mL/kg/hr) is evident at the time of the scheduled second or third dose, do not give until renal function has returned to normal. If the ductus arteriosus remains patent a second course of therapy may be given (doses unchanged).

Some neonatal units use a 6 dose protocol as follows: 100 microgram/kg IV or orally daily for 6 days. In established symptomatic PDA the first dose is given as 200

NOTES

- **Administration IV for the closure of PDA:** reconstitute the vial with 1-2mL of NaCl 0.9% or Water for Injections (1mL of diluent gives a concentration of 100 microgram in 0.1mL; 2mL of diluent gives a concentration of 50 microgram in 0.1mL). Preparations containing glucose must not be used. The indometacin solution may be injected IV over 20 minutes. This recommendation is based on published reports which indicate that there is a transient reduction in cerebral blood flow velocity and cerebral blood flow when the injection is rapidly infused over 5 minutes. A syringe pump which delivers rates of 0.1-0.2mL per hour can be used. With small injection volumes, it is necessary to consider the priming volume of the tubing and flush through with a suitable volume of fluid, following the active injection, given at the same rate.

- Indometacin injection is contra-indicated in established or suspected untreated infection and bleeding disorders.

- Use with caution in patients with renal impairment, or severe liver impairment.

- Avoid in patients with active peptic ulcer disease and in asthmatics with known hypersensitivity to NSAIDs.

- None of the currently available oral or rectal preparations are licensed for use in children. The injection is only licensed for the closure of PDA in premature babies. The oral suspension is available as a 'special' from Eldon Laboratories and a German product may be imported via IDIS; both are unlicensed.

Insulins

- **Vials:** 100 units/mL.
- **Cartridges:** for use with reusable pens.

DOSAGE
Diabetes presenting without ketoacidosis

- **Prefilled disposable pens.**
Not all types of insulin are available in all presentations.

Initial dose: 0.5-0.7 units/kg/day SC; two-thirds of the total dose administered in the morning and one-third in the evening. Administer 30 minutes before meals except if using very short acting insulin, Humalog® (insulin lispro) or NovoRapid® (insulin aspart), when insulin is administered immediately before eating.

Diabetes presenting with ketoacidosis

After starting IV fluids, give an IV infusion of low-dose soluble insulin (0.1units/kg/hour). Adjust according to blood glucose level. See guidelines section of *Medicines for Children*.

Long-term management of diabetes

Insulin dosage and frequency of administration will vary according to clinical circumstances and monitoring of blood sugars.

NOTES

■ Insulin should be stored in the refrigerator, but has a shelf-life of 1 month when stored at room temperature.

■ Insulin should be prescribed by trade name, all parents/patients should be familiar with the brand of insulin they are using.

PREPARATIONS

The insulins listed are classed as human; beef and pork insulins are also available.

Very short acting

Humalog® (*insulin lispro*) (Lilly). Available as vials, prefilled pens & cartridges. Onset of action within 15 minutes. Duration of action approximately 2–5 hours.

NovoRapid® (*insulin aspart*) (Novo Nordisk). Available as vials, prefilled pens & cartridges. Onset of action within 10-20 minutes. Duration of action is

Short acting (soluble)

Human Velosulin® (Novo Nordisk). Available as vials only. Duration of action approximately 8 hours.

Human Actrapid® (Novo Nordisk). Available as vials, prefilled pens, cartridges. Duration of action approximately 8 hours.

Humulin S® (Lilly). Available as vials, prefilled pens, cartridges. Duration of action approximately 12 hours.

Insuman® Rapid (Aventis Pharma). Available as vials, prefilled pens and cartridges. Duration of action 7–9 hours.

Medium acting (isophane)

Human Insulatard®ge (Novo Nordisk). Available as vials, prefilled pens, cartridges. Duration of action approximately 24 hours.

Humulin I® (Lilly). Available as vials, prefilled pens, cartridges. Duration of action approximately 22 hours.

Insuman® Basal (Aventis Pharma). Available as vials, prefilled pens and cartridges. Duration of action 11–20 hours.

Medium acting (insulin zinc suspension)

Human Monotard® (Novo Nordisk). Available as vials only. Duration of action approximately 24 hours.

Humulin Lente® (Lilly). Available as vials only. Duration of action approximately 23 hours.

The list of Insulin preparations continues overleaf

Long acting (crystalline zinc suspension)

Human Ultratard® (Novo Nordisk). Available as vials only. Duration of action approximately 24-28 hours.

PREPARATIONS [continued]
Long acting (crystalline zinc suspension) [continued]

Humulin Zn® (Lilly). Available as vials only. Duration of action approximately 25 hours.

Lantus® (insulin glarine) (Aventis). Available as vials, prefilled pens and cartridges. Duration of action approximately 15-30 hours.

Biphasic (soluble and isophane)
Speed of onset of the combination products is proportional to the amount of soluble insulin.

Human Mixtard® (Novo Nordisk). Available as 10/90, 20/80, 30/70, 40/60 and 50/50 mixtures, in prefilled pens, cartridges. Only the 30/70 and 50/50 mixtures are available in vials. Total duration of action approximately 24 hours. Maximum effect is exerted between 2 and 8 hours after SC injection.

Humulin M® (Lilly). Available as M2, 20/80 in prefilled pens and cartridges; M3 30/70, in vials, prefilled pens and cartridges. M5, 50/50 is only available in vials. Total duration of action is approximately 22 hours, with a peak duration of activity of 4 hours.

Insuman® Comb (Aventis Pharma). Available as 15/85, 25/75 and 50/50 mixtures in prefilled pens, vials and cartridges. Duration of action 12–18 hours. Peak effect is exerted between 2 and 4 hours after SC injection.

Biphasic Insulin Lispro

Humalog® Mix (Lilly). Available as Mix 25 (25% insulin lispro, 75% insulin lispro protamine) in prefilled pens and cartridges and Mix 50 (a 50/50 mix of insulin lispro and insulin lispro protamine) in prefilled pens. They have an onset of action within 15 minutes, peak effect after approximately 1 hour and a duration of action of up to 15 hours.

Biphasic Insulin Aspart

NovoMix®30 (Lilly). Available as 30/70 mixture, in prefilled pens and cartridges. Onset of action will occur within 10 to 20 minutes, peak effect is exerted between 1 and 4 hours and duration of action is up to 24 hours.

- **Aerosol inhaler:** 20 microgram, 40 microgram per actuation.
- **Breath actuated inhaler:** 20 microgram per actuation.
- **Dry powder for inhalation:** 40 microgram.
- **Nebuliser solution:** 250 microgram in 1mL, 500 microgram in 2mL.

DOSAGE

Route	Age				Frequency (times daily)	Notes
	birth–1 month	1 month–2 years	2–12 years	12–18 years		
Inhaled	←	Up to 120 microgram		→	4	RELIEVER For symptom relief only.
Dry powder inhalation	-	-	-	40 microgram (1 capsule)	3-4	RELIEVER For symptom relief only.
Nebulised	25 microgram/kg	<1 year 62.5 microgram	<5 years 125-250 microgram	500 microgram	single dose	Can be repeated every 20-30 minutes in the first 2 hours in acute severe asthma. Reduce dose frequency as clinical improvement occurs.
		>1 year 125-250 microgram	>5years 250-500 microgram		single dose	

NOTES

■ Nebuliser solution can be diluted with NaCl 0.9% or mixed with salbutamol, budesonide or terbutaline nebuliser solutions.

■ Inhalers can be used via Nebuhaler®, Volumatic® or Aerochamber® spacer devices.

■ The doses and dose frequencies stated exceed those recommended by the manufacturers. The dry powder for inhalation is not licensed for use in children.

Iron

■ **Tablets:** ferrous sulphate 200mg (65mg Fe); ferrous fumarate 322mg (100mg Fe); ferrous gluconate 300mg (35mg Fe).

■ **Syrups:** sodium feredetate 27.5mg Fe in 5mL (Sytron®); ferrous glycine sulphate 25mg Fe in 5mL (Plesmet®); ferrous fumarate 45mg Fe in 5mL (Fersamal® and Galfer®).

There are many iron preparations available - for further details and information on injectable iron see *Medicines for Children*.

DOSAGE

Newborn infant

Indication	Route	Age	Frequency	Notes
		birth–1 month	(times daily)	
Prophylaxis of iron deficiency in low birth weight (<2.5 kg), breast-fed infants	Oral	5 mg of elemental iron or 1mL Sytron® elixir	1

1 | Usually started at 28 days postnatal age and continued until mixed feeding is established. There is no good evidence that formula fed babies require further supplementation after discharge (unless they are on Osterprem®). Current practice varies throughout the UK; refer to local policy as doses may differ from those stated. |

DOSAGE

Child

Indication	Route	Age			Frequency	Notes
		1 month–2 years	2–12 years	12–18 years	(times daily)	
Treatment of iron deficiency anaemia	Oral	← 2.5mg/kg → of elemental iron		-	2	
		-		60mg	3	

NOTES

■ Gastro-intestinal side-effects are common: nausea, epigastric pain, diarrhoea, constipation.

■ A positive response to treatment is demonstrated after 6-8 weeks by a rise in haemoglobin of at least 1g/100mL over a month.

■ Products differ in their licensed indications. Check individual product information carefully. Refer to *Medicines for Children* for details. In general, oral liquid iron preparations are licensed for use in all ages.

■ Calculate dose in terms of elemental iron, specifying prescribing in terms of elemental iron or convert the dose to the iron salt preparation required and specify prescribing in terms of the specific salt, with for example, the dose given in mLs.

Isoniazid

■ **Tablets:** 50mg, 100mg.
■ **Oral liquid:** 50mg in 5mL.

■ **Injection:** 25mg in 1mL, 2mL ampoule.

DOSAGE

Route	Age				Frequency (times daily)	Notes
	birth– 1 month	1 month– 2 years	2–12 years	12–18 years		
Oral/IM/IV	5mg/kg	←	10mg/kg (maximum 300mg)	→	1	See guidelines in 2nd Edition *Medicines for Children for Children* for further information. Doses may be doubled in tuberculous meningitis (maximum 500mg).

▯ ◧ ▣ᴿ

NOTES

■ **Administration: IV:** by slow bolus of the undiluted injection.

■ Rate of metabolism of phenytoin, carbamazepine and diazepam may be reduced by isoniazid.

■ Absorption of isoniazid may be reduced by concurrent administration of antacids.

■ ▯ Use with caution in hepatic impairment; monitor hepatic function.

■ ◧ Use with caution in renal impairment; dosage adjustments are generally not necessary until creatinine clearance falls to 10mL/min/1.73m²; such patients may require a dose reduction to maintain trough plasma levels of 1mg/L.

■ ▣ᴿ Licensed for use in all ages with the exception of the oral liquid which is available as a 'special' from several 'specials' manufacturers and as such is unlicensed.

Isoprenaline

▣ᴿ

■ **Injection:** (as hydrochloride) 20 microgram in 1mL, 10mL disposable syringe; (as sulphate) 2.25mg in 2mL ampoule and other strengths available as 'specials'.

DOSAGE

Route	Age				Frequency (times daily)	Notes
	birth– 1 month	1 month– 2 years	2–12 years	12–18 years		
IV infusion	20–300 nanogram/	◄— 20 nanogram/kg/minute – 1microgram/kg/minute —►		1–4 microgram/ minute	continuous	Use the lowest possible effective dose. Doses in terms of hydrochloride salt. 2.25mg isoprenaline sulphate =

NOTES

■ **Administration: IV:** compatible with glucose 5% or NaCl 0.9%. Separate administration of alkaline infusions e.g. sodium bicarbonate is advised. Maximum infusion rate: 1 microgram/kg/minute.

■ Isoprenaline is licensed for use in adults and children with the exception of the 'specials' which are unlicensed.

■ 'Specials' available from various NHS manufacturing units and Martindale Pharmaceuticals Ltd.

Labetalol

■ **Tablets:** 50mg, 100mg, 200mg, 400mg.
■ **Injection:** 5mg in 1mL; 20mL ampoule.

■ **Oral solution:** may be extemporaneously prepared

DOSAGE

Route	Age				Frequency (times daily)	Notes
	birth– 1 month	1 month– 2 years	2–12 years	12–18 years		
IV bolus	–	◄ 250–500 microgram/kg ►		50mg	single dose	Loading dose.
IV infusion	500 microgram/kg/ hour up to a max of 4mg/kg/hour	◄ 1–3mg/kg/hour ►		120 mg/hour	continuous	Start at low dose and titrate according to response, until the blood pressure has been reduced to an acceptable level.

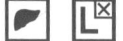

DOSAGE continued

Route	Age				Frequency (times daily)	Notes
	birth–1 month	1 month–2 years	2–12 years	12–18 years		
Oral	–	← 1–2mg/kg →		50–200mg (maximum 300mg)	3–4	

NOTES

■ **Administration: oral:** injection can be given orally with juice. **IV infusion:** infuse in glucose 5% or glucose 4%/NaCl 0.18% at a concentration of 1mg in 1mL. Can be administered undiluted in fluid restricted patients. **IV bolus:** give over at least 1 minute.

■ Avoid in liver disease; stop if liver dysfunction occurs.

■ Avoid in asthma, heart failure and heart block.

■ See propranolol monograph in *Medicines for Children* for further information, re: side effects, interactions etc.

Lactulose

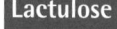

■ **Solution:** 3.1-3.7g in 5mL (depending on the brand).

DOSAGE

Indication	Route	Age			Frequency (times daily)	Notes
		1 month–2 years	2–12 years	12–18 years		
Constipation	Oral	<1 year 2.5mL 1–2 years 5mL	<5 years 5mL 5–10 years 10mL 10–12 years 15mL	15mL	2 2 2	Initial dose. Then adjust to suit patient.
Hepatic encephalopathy	Oral	–	–	30–50mL	3	Initial dose Then adjust the dose to produce 2-3 soft stools a day.

NOTES

■ **Administration:** may be taken with water or other fluids.

■ Relatively ineffective in opioid-induced constipation as primarily an osmotic rather than a stimulant laxative.

■ May take up to 48 hours before effects are obtained.

■ ⎣ᴸ⎦ Hepatic encephalopathy is a licensed indication in adults only.

■ **Tablets:** 25mg, 50mg, 100mg, 200mg.

■ **Tablets (dispersible):** 2mg, 5mg, 25mg, 100mg.

DOSAGE

Indication	Route	Age		Frequency (times daily)	Notes
		2–12 years	**12–18 years**		
When given with sodium valproate (with/ without any anti-epileptics)	Oral	150 microgram/kg*	–	1	Weeks 1 and 2. * If the calculated dose is 2.5–5mg (ie – patients weighing 17–33kg), then 5mg may be taken on alternate days for weeks 1 and 2.
		–	25mg	alternate days	
		300 microgram/kg	25mg	1	Weeks 3 and 4. Total daily dose may be given as two divided doses.
		500 microgram/kg- 2.5 mg/kg (maximum 100mg)	50-100mg	2	<u>Usual target maintenance dose</u> To achieve maintenance increase every 1-2 weeks by: 150 microgram/kg/dose (2-12 years) 12.5-25mg/dose (12-18 years). Total daily dose may be given as a single dose.

Indication	Route	Age		Frequency (times daily)	Notes
		2–12 years	12–18 years		
When given with enzyme inducing anti-epileptics other than sodium valproate	Oral	300 microgram/kg	–	2	Weeks 1 and 2.
		–	25mg	2	
		600 microgram/kg	50mg	2	Weeks 3 and 4
		2.5-7.5mg/kg (maximum 200mg)	100-200mg	2	Usual target maintenance dose To achieve maintenance increase every 1-2 weeks by: 600 microgram/kg/dose (2-12 years) 50mg/dose (12-18 years).
Monotherapy	Oral	–	25mg	1	Weeks 1 and 2
		–	50mg	1	Weeks 3 and 4 Total daily dose may be given as two divided doses.
		–	100-200mg	1	Usual target maintenance dose To achieve maintenance increase the daily dose by 50-100mg every 1-2 weeks. Total daily dose may be given as two divided doses.

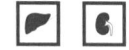

NOTES

- **Administration:** dispersible tablets are to be chewed or dissolved in water. Tablets can be crushed and mixed with syrup or jam just before administration.

- Reduce initial doses in liver disease and titrate to response.

- Use with caution in renal failure.

- Drug interactions can occur with other anticonvulsant drugs e.g. carbamazepine, phenytoin, phenobarbital and primidone may enhance the metabolism of lamotrigine and increase dose requirement.

- Not licensed for infants and children <2 years of age. Not licensed for monotherapy <12 years of age.

Levothyroxine (thyroxine) sodium

- **Tablets:** 25 microgram, 50 microgram, 100 microgram.
- **Capsules**: 12.5 microgram.
- **Oral liquid**: may be extemporaneously prepared.

DOSAGE

Route	Age				Frequency (times daily)	Notes
	birth–1 month	1 month–2 years	2–12 years	12–18 years		
Oral	10–15	5–10	5	50–100	1	

NOTES

- Infants may be treated with crushed tablets, allowing dosage increments of 12.5 micrograms. Treatment aims in congenital hypothyroidism are to correct free thyroxine to >20pmol/L within 2 weeks, and thyroid stimulating hormone (TSH) to <10 milliunits/L within 4 weeks. Thyroid function should be monitored at 2 weekly intervals until target levels, followed by diminishing frequency guided by progress and compliance.

- In older children, dosage changes are made in increments of 25 micrograms and are guided by tests at 4-8 weeks until normal adult ranges are reached, after which biochemical monitoring may be reduced to 6-12 monthly

- Levothyroxine sodium is licensed for use in all ages with the exception of the oral liquid which needs to be extemporaneously prepared and is therefore unlicensed, and the 12.5 microgram capsules which are available as a 'special' from Martindale.

Lidocaine (lignocaine) hydrochloride

- **Injection:** 0.5% (5mg in 1mL), 10mL ampoule. 1% (10mg in 1mL), 2mL, 5mL, 10mL and 20mL ampoule; 10mL disposable syringe. 2% (20mg in 1mL), 2mL, 5mL, 10mL and 20mL ampoule; 5mL disposable syringe.

- **Injection (with adrenaline):** 0.5% with adrenaline (epinephrine) 1 in 200,000, 20mL vial. 1% with adrenaline (epinephrine) 1 in 200,000, 20mL vial. 2% with adrenaline (epinephrine) 1 in 200,000, 20mL vial.

- **Infusion:** 0.1% (1mg/mL) or 0.2% (2mg/mL) in glucose 5%, 500mL container.

- **Dental injection:** a large variety of lidocaine injections, plain or with adrenaline (epinephrine) or noradrenaline (norepinephrine), is available in dental cartridges

- **Gel:** 1%, 2%; 15mL tube.

- **Gel:** 2% with chlorhexidine gluconate 0.25%, 6mL and 11mL disposable syringes.

- **Ointment:** 5%; 15g tube.

- **Pump spray:** 10%; 50mL bottle.

- **Topical solution:** 4%; 30mL bottle

DOSAGE

Indication	Route	Age				Frequency	Notes
		birth–1 month	1 month–2 years	2–12 years	12–18 years		
Anti-arrhythmic	IV bolus	← 500 microgram/kg - 1mg/kg → then			50–100mg then infusion (as shown below)	single dose	<u>Loading dose</u> In the 12-18 year age group give 50mg in lighter patients or those whose circulation is severely impaired.
	IV infusion	← 10–50 microgram/kg/**minute** → (600 microgram/kg/hour – 3mg/kg/hour)			4mg/minute for 30 minutes then 2mg/minute for 2 hours then 1 mg/minute reducing concentration further if infusion is continued beyond	continuous	<u>Maintenance dosing:</u> ECG monitoring with infusion.

Indication	Route	Age				Frequency	Notes
		birth–1 month	1 month–2 years	2–12 years	12–18 years		
VF or pulseless tachycardia	IV/IO	←———— 1mg/kg ————→ (maximum dose 100mg)			50-100mg	single dose	Repeat every 5 minutes if needed to a total maximum of 3mg/kg. In the 12-18 year age group give 50mg in lighter patients or those whose circulation is severely impaired.
Local anaesthetic	Local infiltration	←———— up to 3mg/kg ————→			up to 200mg	single dose	Not more often than every 4 hours. Use fine needles (27-29) gauge.
	Intra-urethral	←———— 3-4mg/kg ————→				single dose	Prior to urinary catheterisation. Warm the solution to body temperature and inject it very slowly to reduce local stinging.
Dental	Topical	–	Apply sparingly to dried oral mucosa at the proposed site of injection.			single dose	2% gel.
	Infiltration	–	←———— 1mL ————→			single dose	2% solution with adrenaline (epinephrine) 1:80,000.
	Nerve block	–	←———— 1.5-2mL ————→			single dose	

NOTES

■ **Administration: IV:** compatible with glucose 5% or NaCl 0.9%.

■ Avoid, or reduce dose, in severe liver disease.

■ Use as an antiarrhythmic is unlicensed. Local anaesthetic and dental use licensed in children and adults.

■ Contra-indicated in AV block, sino atrial disorders, severe myocardial depression and porphyria.

■ Local anaesthetics should not be given into inflamed or infected tissues.

■ Great care must be taken to avoid intravascular injection. Careful surveillance for toxic effects is necessary for the first 30 minutes following oral injection.

Lidocaine (lignocaine) & prilocaine cream-Emla®

■ **Cream:** lidocaine 2.5% and prilocaine 2.5%, 5g and 30g tubes – Emla®

DOSAGE

Indication	Route	Age				Frequency	Notes
		birth–1 month	1 month–2 years	2–12 years	12–18 years		
Minor procedures e.g. vene-	Topical	Not recommended	Approx. 2g for a minimum of 1 hour and a maximum of 5 hours (under an occlusive dressing)			single dose	Smaller amounts may be adequate for small children and infants.

DOSAGE continued

Indication	Route	Age				Frequency	Notes
		birth–1 month	1 month–2 years	2–12 years	12–18 years		
Procedures to larger areas e.g. split skin grafting	Topical	Not recommended	Approx. 1.5 –3g per 10cm² for a minimum of 2 hours and a maximum of 5 hours (under an occlusive dressing)			single dose	Smaller amounts may be adequate for small children and infants. Not adequate for heel prick sampling.

NOTES

■ **Administration: Topical:** analgesic efficiency may decline if the cream is applied for longer than 5 hours. Procedures on intact skin should begin soon after the removal of the cream. Duration of analgesia after an application of time 1-2 hours is at least 2 hours after removal of the dressing.

■ Not to be applied to wounds, mucous membranes, areas of atopic dermatitis and genital mucosa in children. Avoid use near eyes or middle ear.

■ Although systemic absorption is low, caution should be exercised in patients with anaemia, congenital or acquired methaemoglobinaemia or on concurrent therapy known to produce such conditions.

■ Licensed for >1 year of age.

L^R

■ **Capsules:** 2mg.   ■ **Syrup:** 1mg in 5mL.

DOSAGE

Route/ indication	Age			Frequency (times daily)	Notes
	1 month–2 years	2–12 years	12–18 years		
Oral/ Chronic diarrhoea e.g. short bowel syndrome	<u><1 year</u> 200 microgram/kg <u>1–2 years</u> 100–200 microgram/kg	As for 1–2 years	2–4mg	30 minutes before feeds 3–4	Doses of up to 2mg/kg/**day** have occasionally been required <1 year.
Oral/ acute diarrhoea	Not recommended for acute diarrhoea in children.		4mg then 2mg	initial dose after each loose stool	Usual total daily dose of 6–8 mg. Maximum daily dose 16mg. Up to 5 days only

NOTES

■ L^R Treatment of chronic diarrhoea is only licensed in adults. Not licensed for use in children less than 4 years of age for acute diarrhoea (but note that it is not recommended for acute diarrhoea in children even though it is licensed)!

■ If intoxication is suspected, naloxone may be given as an antidote.

■ **Tablets:** 1mg, 2.5mg.
■ **Suspension:** several strengths available as 'specials'.

■ **Injection:** 4mg in 1mL.

DOSAGE

Indication	Route	Age				Frequency	Notes
		birth–1 month	1 month–2 years	2–12 years	12–18 years		
Pre-medication	Oral	–	← 50–100 microgram/kg → (maximum 4mg)		1–4mg	single dose	Give at least one hour before surgery. Round to the nearest 500 microgram.
Pre-medication	IV/IM	–	← 50–100 microgram/kg → (maximum 4mg)			single dose	IV give 30–45 minutes before surgery. IM give 1–1½ hours before surgery. IV is the preferred parenteral route.
Status epilepticus	IV Rectal Sublingual	← 100 microgram/kg → (maximum 4mg)			4mg	single dose	Generally given as a single dose; may be repeated once if initial dose is ineffective. Limited experience in neonates.

NOTES

■ **Administration: IV/IM:** Injection should usually be diluted with an equal volume of NaCl 0.9% or Water for Injections before administration. IV injections should be given at a rate not exceeding 2mg/min into a large vein.

■ Avoid in patients with pre-existing CNS depression or coma, or respiratory failure.

■ **C** In severe renal impairment use 50% of dose (increased cerebral sensitivity). Dose reduction is not necessary in mild to moderate renal impairment.

■ **L** Dose reduction is not usually necessary in liver disease. Caution in severe liver disease; may precipitate coma.

■ **LS** Tablets licensed in children from 5 years of age for premedication. Injection not licensed < 12 years of age for premedication. Injection licensed in children for treatment of status epilepticus. Rectal administration of the injection is unlicensed. Suspensions are unlicensed preparations.

■ Suspensions available from BCM Specials.

NOTES

- **Administration:** Powder from capsule may be dispersed in water, milk or orange juice.

- Clearance is reduced significantly and half-life prolonged in cirrhotic patients. Relevance in terms of dose adjustments in patients with liver disease is unclear.

- Immediate release formulations may be more effective in inducing sleep, sustained-release formulations may be better for maintenance of sleep. Melatonin treatment is likely to be more successful when combined with strict environmental sleep structuring. It may be possible to withdraw the drug after 2-3 months when a regular sleep pattern has been established.

- UL All preparations are available on a named patient basis (from IDIS World Medicines or Penn Pharmaceuticals) and as such are unlicensed.

Meropenem

- Injection: (as trihydrate salt) 500mg and 1g vials.

DOSAGE
Newborn infant (birth to 1 month)

Route	Postnatal age	Dose	Frequency (times daily)	Notes
IV	<7 days	20 mg/kg	2	Double dose in meningitis or severe infection.
	>7 days	20 mg/kg	3	

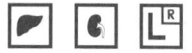

Child

Route	Age			Frequency (times daily)	Notes
	1 month-2 years	2-12 years	12-18 years		
IV	←	10mg/kg	→	3	UTI, gynaecological, skin and skin structure infections. Maximum single dose 500mg.
	←	20mg/kg	→	3	Pneumonia, peritonitis, neutropenia, septicaemia. Maximum single dose 1g.
	←	40mg/kg	→	3	Meningitis, life threatening infections and cystic fibrosis patients. Maximum single dose 2g.

 Dose adjustment in renal impairment

Creatinine clearance (mL/min/1.73m²)	Dose	Dosage interval
25-50	100%	12 hours
10-25	50%	12 hours
<10	50%	24 hours

NOTES

■ **Administration: IV:** administered by slow IV injection over 5 minutes or by IV infusion over 20-30 minutes. Each 250mg displaces 0.22mL of water on reconstitution. For slow IV injection a concentration of 50mg in 1mL should be used. May be further diluted with glucose 5% or 10%, or NaCl

0.9% to provide a solution between 1-50mg in 1mL for IV infusion.

■ 🔲 Monitor LFTs carefully in patients with pre-existing liver disease.

■ 🔲 Licensed for >3 months of age.

Methylphenidate hydrochloride (controlled drug)

🔲

■ **Tablets:** 5mg, 10mg, 20mg (all scored).

■ **Tablets (modified release):** 18mg, 36mg.

DOSAGE

Route	Age		Frequency (times daily)	Notes
	2-12 years	12-18 years		
Oral	≥6 years 5mg	5mg	1 or 2	<u>Initial dose</u> Increase if necessary by weekly increments of 5–10mg daily. Maximum of 60mg **per day** given in 2-4 divided doses.
Oral (m/r)	≥6 years 18mg	18mg	1 (morning)	<u>Initial dose</u> Increase if necessary by weekly increments of 18mg daily, according to response. Maximum of 54mg daily.

NOTES

■ **Administration:** Normal release tablets may be halved, but unreliable dose if quartered. If anorexia is a problem give dose after breakfast and lunch. If rebound hyperactivity occurs in the latter part of the day the dose can be given in further divided doses. Methylphenidate can cause insomnia so the last dose should not usually be given any later than 4pm.

■ Licensed for use in children ≥ 6 years of age.

■ Treatment must be under the supervision of a specialist in childhood behavioural disorders and should be part of a comprehensive treatment programme for ADHD.

Methylprednisolone

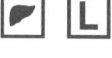

■ **Injection:** 40mg, 125mg, 500mg, 1g, 2g vials.

DOSAGE

Indication	Route	Age			Frequency (times daily)	Notes
		1 month–2 years	2–12 years	12–18 years		
Severe JIA, connective tissue diseases	IV	←	30mg/kg	→	once daily	Give daily for 3 days. Maximum 1g/day.
Graft rejection	IV	←	10–20mg/kg	→	once daily	

Indication	Route	Age			Frequency	Notes
		1 month–2 years	2–12 years	12–18 years	(times daily)	
Demyelinating disorders	IV	← 500mg →		1g	once daily	

NOTES

- **Administration: IV:** give over at least 30 minutes. It may be diluted with NaCl 0.9% or glucose 5%.

- Prophylactic antacid administration may be required.

- If a patient is receiving oral steroids then these are usually stopped on the days that methylprednisolone is given.

- Use is contra-indicated in patients with systemic infection, unless specific anti-infective therapy is used.

- Live vaccines should not be given to patients receiving immunosuppressive doses of steroids.

- Dosage may have to be reduced in patients with hepatic impairment. The lowest effective dose should be used.

Metoclopramide hydrochloride

- **Tablets:** 5mg, 10mg.
- **Syrup/oral solution:** 5mg in 5mL.
- **Paediatric liquid:** 1mg in 1mL.
- **Injection:** 5mg in 1mL; 2mL ampoule.

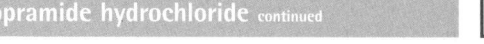

DOSAGE

Route	Age				Frequency (times daily)	Notes
	birth– 1 month	1 month– 2 years	2–12 years	12–18 years		
Oral, IM, slow IV bolus	← 100 microgram/kg →				2–3	Higher doses may be needed with chemotherapy but <12 years of age total daily dose should not exceed 500 microgram/kg (maximum 10mg) per day. Can be given more frequently with chemotherapy.
				<60kg 5mg	3	
				>60kg 10mg	3	

NOTES

■ **Administration: IV:** as a slow bolus injection over at least 5 minutes or for doses over 10mg at a suggested concentration of 200 micrograms per mL over 15-30 minutes. Dilute in NaCl 0.9% or glucose 5% if required. For diagnostic procedures, IV dose is given 15-20 minutes before procedure.

■ In mild to moderate renal impairment use 75% of a dose and in severe impairment 25-50% of a dose.

■ Reduce dose in severe liver disease.

■ Extrapyramidal side-effects can be treated with an anticholinergic e.g. benztropine.

■ Licensed for use in adults and children (tablets only licensed ≥ 15 years of age); however, use in patients <20 years of age should be restricted to: prophylaxis/treatment of vomiting associated with chemotherapy/radiotherapy, intractable vomiting of known cause, premedication for jejunal biopsy and small bowel intubation to assist passage through the pylorus, palliative care as a prokinetic for chronic or opioid-induced constipation.

- **Tablets:** 200mg, 400mg, 500mg.
- **Oral suspension:** 200mg in 5mL.
- **IV infusion:** 5mg in 1mL, 20mL ampoule, 100mL bag (in NaCl 0.9%).
- **Suppositories:** 125mg, 250mg, 500mg, 1g.

DOSAGE
Newborn infant

Route	Age	Frequency	Notes
	birth–1 month	(times daily)	
IV	15mg/kg	single dose	Loading dose followed 24 hours later by twice daily dosing as shown.
	7.5mg/kg	2	Oral therapy may be used when absorption considered normal.

Child

Route	Age			Frequency	Notes
	1 month–2 years	2–12 years	12–18 years	(times daily)	
Oral	← 7.5mg/kg → (maximum 400mg)		400mg	3	Anaerobic infections. Disorders of propionate metabolism. Oral route has excellent bioavailability; reserve IV route for serious infections or when oral route is not available.
IV	← 7.5mg/kg → (maximum 500mg)		500mg	3	

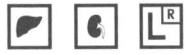

Child continued

Route	Age			Frequency (times daily)	Notes
	1 month–2 years	2–12 years	12–18 years		
Rectal	DOSE BY WEIGHT		1g	3	Anaerobic infections
	7.5mg/kg				Substitute oral therapy as soon as possible. ie after 3 days rectal therapy,
	or DOSE BY AGE				change to oral therapy or reduce rectal frequency to twice daily.
	≤1 year	1–5 years	5–12 years			
	125mg	250mg	500mg	3	
Oral	40mg/kg			1	Giardiasis for 3 days.
	(maximum 2g)				
Oral	5mg/kg		300mg	3	Trichomoniasis for 7 days.
			or		
			400mg	2	For 7 days.
			or		
			2g	single dose	
Oral	10mg/kg		400–800mg	3	Amoebiasis – for 5–10 days.
					Balantidiasis – for 5 days.

Child continued

Route	Age			Frequency (times daily)	Notes
	1 month–2 years	2–12 years	12–18 years		
Oral for *H. pylori*	>1 year 100mg	2–6 years 100mg	400mg	3	Treatment for 14 days with amoxicillin and omeprazole.
		6–12 years 200mg		3	
	>1 year 100mg	2–6 years 100mg	400mg	2	Treatment for 14 days with clarithromycin and omeprazole.
		6–12 years 200mg		2	

NOTES

■ **Administration: oral:** tablets should be swallowed whole with or after food. Suspension should be administered one hour before food. **IV:** infusion over 20-30 minutes. Maximum rate 25mg per minute. May be diluted in glucose 5%, NaCl 0.9%, glucose 4%/NaCl 0.18% or potassium infusions (20 or 40mmol/L).

■ C Increase dose interval to 12 hourly in severe renal impairment (creatinine clearance <20mL/min/1.73m²).

■ Reduce dose in severe liver disease. Avoid in hepatic encephalopathy.

■ L 125mg and 250mg suppositories are available as 'specials' from the manufacturing unit of the Royal Hallamshire Hospital and are unlicensed preparations. Not licensed for use in neonates. Infusion not licensed for use <1 year of age.

■ **Injection:** 10mg in 2mL; 10mg in 5mL; 1mg in 1mL, 50mL vial; 5mg in 1mL, 2mL, 5mL, 10mL and 18mL ampoule.

■ **Oral solution:** 2.5mg in 1mL.
■ **Buccal liquid:** 10mg in 1mL.

DOSAGE

Newborn infant

Indication	Route	Age	Frequency	Notes
		birth–1 month		
Sedation	IV infusion	1 microgram/kg/minute for the first 24 hours then decrease to 500 nanogram/kg/minute in babies <33 weeks postconceptional age to avoid accumulation.	continuous	Can be used for up to 4 days with apparent safety in the ventilated newborn baby.

Child

Indication	Route	Age			Frequency	Notes
		1 month–2 years	2–12 years	12–18 years		
Premedication	IM	← 70–100 microgram/kg →			single dose	Administer 30–60 minutes prior to surgery. Monitor from time of administration.
	Oral	← 500 microgram/kg (maximum dose 15mg) →			single dose	
Sedation for procedures	IV bolus	–		2mg	single dose	If after 2 minutes sedation is not adequate, incremental doses of 500 microgram – 1mg can be given. Doses >5mg are rarely needed.
	IV bolus or IM	← 50–100 microgram/kg →		–	single dose	Doses up to 300 microgram/kg may sometimes be needed.
	Oral	← 500 microgram/kg (maximum dose 15mg) →			single dose	
	Rectal	← 500–750 microgram/kg →			single dose	
	Intranasal	← 200–300 microgram/kg →			single dose	Half the dose should be given into each nostril.
Sedation in intensive care	IV bolus (over 3–5 minutes)	← 30–300 microgram/kg →			single dose	This may not be needed if the patient is already receiving morphine or is sedated post-op. Reduce the dose in hypovolaemia, vaso-constriction and hypothermia. Low doses may also be adequate if the patient is also receiving an opiate. Adjust according to response.
		then				
	IV infusion	← 500 nanogram/kg/minute–3.3 microgram/kg/minute →			continuous	

Child continued

Indication	Route	Age			Frequency	Notes
		1 month–2 years	2–12 years	12–18 years		
Induction of anaesthesia	Slow IV bolus	–	≥7 years 150 microgram/kg	200–300 microgram/kg	single dose	In adults the dose should be titrated against individual response. Young fit unpremedicated patients may require at least 300 microgram/kg. Those premedicated with an opiate usually only require a dose of 200 microgram/kg.
Status epilepticus	IV bolus	← 150-200 microgram/kg →			single dose	Initial bolus. Follow with infusion as below.
	IV infusion	← 1 microgram/kg/minute → increasing by 1 microgram/kg/minute every 15 minutes until the seizure stops Maximum of 5 microgram/kg/minute			continuous	Start with the initial bolus above before commencing the infusion. Not yet an established drug in this area. Most experience in paediatric intensive care units.
	Buccal/ intranasal	DOSE BY WEIGHT <6 months 300 microgram/kg DOSE BY AGE >6 months 2.5mg	1-4 years 5mg 5-9 years 7.5mg >10 years 10mg	10mg	single dose single dose single dose	Buccal administration is the preferred route over intranasal administration.

NOTES

■ **Administration: rectal, intranasal:** the injection may be given buccally intranasally and rectally. **Oral:** if the injection is used orally the bitter taste may be disguised by apple or blackcurrant juice or chocolate sauce, however, oral liquids are available.

■ Caution in patients with respiratory failure.

■ Drug interactions: erythromycin and other macrolide antibiotics, cimetidine, itraconazole, ketoconazole and fluconazole all enhance the effect of midazolam.

■ Ⓛ Hypnovel® 10mg/2mL is licensed in children for sedation in intensive care units, premedication before induction of anaesthesia in children and conscious sedation before and during diagnostic or therapeutic procedures with or without local anaesthesia. Other routes and indications are not licensed. The oral and buccal solutions are available as 'specials' from Special Products Limited; they are unlicensed products.

Montelukast

■ **Tablets (chewable):** 4mg, 5mg.

■ **Tablets:** 10mg.

DOSAGE

Route	Age		Frequency (times daily)	Notes
	2–12 years	**12–18 years**		
Oral	2–5 years 4mg	12–14 years 5mg	1	At bedtime
	6–12 years 5mg	15–18 years 10mg	1	

NOTES

■ Ⓛ Licensed for use ≥2 years of age. Not licensed for monotherapy and should be added to inhaled anti-inflammatory treatments (e.g. inhaled corticosteroids).

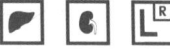

- **Tablets:** 10mg, 20mg, 50mg.
- **Tablets/capsules (modified release):** 5mg, 10mg, 15mg, 20mg, 30mg, 50mg, 60mg, 90mg, 100mg, 120mg, 150mg, 200mg.
- **Oral solution:** 10mg in 5mL, 100mL, 300mL, 500mL bottles, 5mL unit dose vial; 30mg in 5mL, 5mL unit dose vial; 100mg in 5mL, 30mL, 120mL bottles.

- **Granules for oral suspension (modified release):** 20mg, 30mg, 60mg, 100mg and 200mg per sachet.
- **Injection:** 10mg, 15mg, 20mg & 30mg in 1mL; 1mL and 2mL ampoules; 10mg in 1mL in a 1mL disposable syringe. Other strengths of injection are available as 'specials'.
- **Suppositories:** 5mg (available as 'special'), 10mg, 15mg, 20mg, 30mg.

DOSAGE

Newborn infant

Route	Age	Frequency	Notes
	birth–1 month	(times daily)	
Slow IV bolus	40–100 microgram/kg	6 hourly	Give over at least 5–10 minutes.
IV infusion (preterm)	25–50 microgram/kg then 5 microgram/kg/hour	single dose continuous	Loading dose.
IV infusion (term)	50–100microgram/kg then 10–20 microgram/kg/hour	single dose continuous	Loading dose. Doses up to a maximum of 40 microgram/kg/hour have been used.

Note: Newborn infants show an increased susceptibility to respiratory depression and therefore appropriate monitoring should be undertaken. Respiratory support should be available for non-ventilated patients.

Child: premedication and analgesia for acute/post-operative pain

Route	Age			Frequency (times daily)	Notes
	1 month–2 years	2–12 years	12–18 years		
IM/SC Injection	100–200 microgram/kg	200 microgram/kg	5–20mg	≤6 months up to 4 times in 24 hours	Respiratory monitoring is mandatory. Give IV over at least 5–10 minutes. ≤1 year use the lower stated dose and consider oxygen saturation monitoring
IV bolus	← 100–200 microgram/kg →		2.5–10mg	>6 months up to 6 times in 24 hours	
IV infusion	← 10–30 microgram/kg/hour → ≤6 months initial rate is 10 microgram/kg/hour >6 months initial rate is 20 microgram/kg/hour			continuous	Use IV bolus as loading dose first.
SC infusion	1–3 months 10 microgram/kg/hour >3 months 20 microgram/kg/hour	← 20 microgram/kg/hour →		continuous	Use 24 gauge cannula over deltoid or abdominal wall. Change rate and change sites every 48–72 hours.

Note: For patient controlled analgesia follow local hospital protocols.

Analgesia and sedation in ventilated and other ITU patients: use IV bolus and infusion doses as shown in the table above as loading and maintenance doses.

⬛ Dose adjustment in renal impairment – in renal failure use 75% of dose if creatinine clearance is 10-50mL/min/1.73m^2 and 50% if it is <10mL/min/1.73m^2.

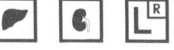
Chronic pain/palliative care

Route	Age			Frequency	Notes
	1 month–2 years	2–12 years	12–18 years	(times daily)	
Oral or rectal	<u><1 year</u> 80 microgram/kg <u>>1 year</u> 200–400 microgram/kg	200–500 microgram/kg	10–15mg	up to 6 times in 24 hours	Starting doses which should be reviewed regularly and adjusted according to the patient's response (see note below table). Doses for relief of dyspnoea in palliative care approximately 50% of those used for analgesia.
SC/IM	150–200 microgram/kg	200 microgram/kg	5–20 mg	up to 6 times in 24 hours	Use with caution if poor peripheral perfusion. Avoid IM injections if possible. Use SC/IM cannula placed under GA or topical LA.

Increase dose in increments of 50% initially until optimum dosages are achieved. Transfer to modified release preparation can then be made. Dose of modified release morphine equals total 24 hour requirement divided by 2 and given 12 hourly or total requirement given once daily depending on product selected. One sixth of daily requirement can be prescribed as oral liquid or non-modified release preparation for control of breakthrough pain. Diamorphine is preferred parenterally because of its higher solubility. Oral morphine 3mg ≡ oral diamorphine 2mg ≡ subcutaneous diamorphine 1mg.

NOTES

■ **Administration: oral:** tablets may be halved. Modified release preparations should not be chewed or crushed. **Parenteral:** injection is stable for at least 24 hours when diluted in glucose 5% or NaCl 0.9%. It is recommended that preservative – free morphine injections be used if possible for continuous infusion to decrease the incidence of phlebitis.

■ Avoid in acute respiratory depression and paralytic ileus.

- Use with caution in raised intra-cranial pressure, head injury or biliary colic.

- Naloxone may be used as an antidote.

- Avoid or reduce dose in liver disease – may precipitate coma.

- Licensing varies depending on the preparation – see *Medicines for Children* for details.

Multivitamins

- **Capsules, tablets, oral drops:** see tables for details.

DOSAGE

Preparation	Age				Frequency (times daily)	Notes
	birth–1 month	1 month–2 years	2–12 years	12–18 years		
Abidec drops *0.6 mL contains:* Vitamin A 1333 units Vitamin D 400 units	0.3mL	≤1year 0.3mL >1 year 0.6mL	← 0.6 mL →		1 1	Supplement for prevention of deficiency states.
Vitamin C 40mg B vitamins	0.6mL	0.6mL	-		1	Premature babies. Dependent on feed - seek dietitians advice.

Preparation	Age				Frequency (times daily)	Notes
	birth– 1 month	1 month– 2 years	2–12 years	12–18 years		
<u>Dalivit drops</u> *0.6 mL contains:* Vitamin A 5000 units Vitamin D 400 units	–	≤1 year 0.3mL ⟵ ≥1 year 0.6 mL	0.6 mL	⟶	1 1	Supplement for prevention of deficiency states.
Vitamin C 50mg B vitamins	–	≤1year 0.6mL ⟵ ≥1 year 1mL	1mL	⟶	1 1	Cystic fibrosis supplement.
<u>Children's</u> Vitamin drops *(DOH)* *0.2mL contains:*	0.2mL	–	–	–	1	Deficiency of prematurity in babies <2.5kg. Continue until on full milk feeds at home.
Vitamin A 1000 units Vitamin D 400 units Vitamin C 30mg	0.4mL	–	–	–	1	Bronchopulmonary dysplasia require extra vitamin A.

Preparation	Age				Frequency (times daily)	Notes
	birth–1 month	1 month–2 years	2–12 years	12–18 years		
Multivitamins BPC *each capsule or tablet contains:* Vitamin A 2500 units Vitamin D 300 units Vitamin C 15mg B vitamins	–	← 1 capsule or tablet →		2 capsules or tablets	1	Supplement for prevention of deficiency states.
	–	2 capsules or tablets	◄2–3 capsules or tablets►		1	Cystic fibrosis supplement.

Ketovite® preparations given by the oral route.

Preparation	Age			Frequency (times daily)	Notes
	1 month– 2 years	2–12 years	12–18 years		
Ketovite liquid *5mL contains:* Vitamin A 2500 units Vitamin D 400 units Choline chloride 150mg Vitamin B₁₂ 12.5microgram	←	5mL liquid	→	1	Tablets and liquid must both be given for complete supplementation.
Ketovite tablets *Each tablet contains:* Thiamine 1mg Riboflavine 1mg Pyridoxine 330 microgram Vitamin C 16.6mg Vitamin E 5mg Nicotinamide 3.3mg Calcium pantothenate 1.16mg Biotin 170 microgram Folic acid 250 microgram Inositol 50mg	←	1 tablet	→	3	

NOTES

■ **Administration:** Ketovite® tablets may be crushed if necessary. Ketovite® liquid can be mixed with milk, cereal or fruit juice. Cystic fibrosis patients who are pancreatic enzyme insufficient should administer vitamin supplements with food and pancreatic enzymes.

■ [L] All presentations are licensed for use in children but the cystic fibrosis doses given here are unlicensed.

■ Cystic fibrosis patients should have serum concentrations of Vitamins A and D monitored at least annually and supplements adjusted accordingly.

■ **Injection:** 400 microgram in 1mL, 1mL ampoule and pre-filled syringe; 20 microgram in 1mL, 2mL ampoule.

DOSAGE

Newborn infant

Route	Age		Frequency	Notes
	birth–1 month			
IV bolus, IM or SC	← 10 microgram/kg →		single dose	May be repeated using doses up to 100 microgram/kg as required, at 2–3 minute intervals.
IV infusion	← 5–20 microgram/kg/hour →		continuous	
IM	← 100 microgram/kg →		single dose	Use 400 microgram/mL naloxone preparation. Gradual onset of action (3–4 minutes) but the effect is sustained for >24 hours.

☐ Do not administer to newborns whose mother's are suspected of narcotic abuse, as a withdrawal syndrome may be precipitated.

☐ Always establish and maintain adequate ventilation before administration of naloxone.

☐ Naloxone is specifically indicated for the reversal of respiratory depression in a newborn infant whose mother has received narcotics within 4 hours of delivery. It is generally preferred to give an IM injection for a prolonged effect.

Child

Route	Age			Frequency	Notes
	1 month–2 years	2–12 years	12–18 year		
IV bolus	← 10 microgram/kg →		10 microgram/kg (max. 800 microgram)	single dose	Initial dose followed by a higher dose if no response.
	then ← 100 microgram/kg → (maximum 2mg)		then 2mg	single dose	Repeat doses as necessary to maintain opioid reversal. Observe for recurrence of CNS and respiratory depression.
IV infusion	← 5–20 microgram/kg/hour →		infuse a solution of 4 microgram/mL at a rate adjusted according to response.	continuous	

NOTES

■ **Administration:** may be given IV, IM, SC or by the intraosseous route.
IV infusion: a continuous infusion may be given when toxicity occurs with long acting opioids. Infusion concentration 2mg in 500mL glucose 5% or NaCl 0.9% i.e. 4 microgram in 1mL.

■ If no response after second dose of naloxone, diagnosis of opioid-induced toxicity should be questioned.

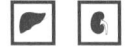

■ **Tablets:** 250mg, 500mg.
■ **Tablets (enteric coated):** 250mg, 375mg, 500mg.

■ **Suspension:** 125mg in 5mL.
■ **Suppositories:** 500mg.

DOSAGE

Route	Age			Frequency (times daily)	Notes
	1 month–2 years	2–12 years	12–18 years		
Oral/rectal	←	5–10mg/kg	→	2	Maximum 1g/day.
Oral	←	10–20mg/kg	→	2	In severe disease. Doses greater than 10mg/kg twice daily not to be used long-term. (Use for a few weeks only).

NOTES

■ **Administration: oral:** enteric coated tablets must be swallowed whole and they may be taken on an empty stomach. Plain tablets may be crushed or chewed and these, and the suspension, should be taken with or after food to minimise gastrointestinal complaints.

■ Use with caution in patients with renal impairment, monitoring serum creatinine and/or creatinine clearance. Avoid use in those with a creatinine clearance <20mL/min/1.73m^2.

■ Use with caution in patients with severe liver impairment.

■ Avoid in patients with active peptic ulcer disease and in asthmatics with known hypersensitivity to NSAIDs.

■ JIA is the only licensed indication for naproxen in children; age/weight licensing restrictions vary depending on the preparation (see *Medicines for Children* for details).

■ Suppository and suspension available from !DIS World Medicines.

■ **Injection:** aqueous solution of netilmicin sulphate 15mg in 1.5mL, 50mg in 1mL, 100mg in 1mL, 150mg in 1.5mL, 200mg in 2mL, expressed as netilmicin base.

DOSAGE

Many dose regimens exist; those outlined below are generally accepted initial doses and dose adjustments should be made in the light of serum concentration measurement.

Divided daily dose regimen

Newborn infant

Route	Birth – 1 month	Frequency	Notes
IV	3mg/kg	12 hourly	Increase to 8 hourly for term neonates >1 week old. Monitor after the third dose aiming for a 1 hour post dose (peak) of 8-12mg/L and a trough level of <3mg/L.

Prolongation of the dosage interval is recommended in newborn infants presenting with PDA, prolonged hypoxia or concurrent treatment with indometacin.

Extended dosing regimen

Newborn infant

Route	Postconceptional age	Dose	Dose frequency	Notes
IV	<32 weeks	6mg/kg	36 hourly	Plasma samples usually taken around the third dose aiming for a pre dose (trough) level of <3mg/L. If there is no change in the dosage regimen or renal function repeat levels every 3-4 days.
	>32 weeks	6mg/kg	24 hourly	

Postconceptional age = gestational plus postnatal age.

Child

Divided daily dose regimen

Route	Age			Frequency (times daily)	Notes
	1 month–2 years	2–12 years	12–18 years		
IV or IM	2.5mg/kg →		2mg/kg	3	Monitor after the third dose aiming for a 1 hour post dose (peak) of 8–12mg/L and a pre dose (trough) level of <3mg/L
Intra-peritoneal	concentrations of 7.5–10mg/L in peritoneal dialysis fluid without elevation of serum levels				

In patients with impaired renal function, dosage and/or frequency of administration must be adjusted in response to serum drug concentrations and the extent of renal impairment. There are various methods to determine dosage and a wide variation in dosage recommendations. See SPC for manufacturers' recommendations.

Child

Single daily dose regimen

Route	Age			Frequency (times daily)	Notes
	1 month–2 years	2–12 years	12–18 years		
IV	← 7.5mg/kg →			1	Plasma levels usually taken at 18–24 hours after the first dose. Aiming for a level of <1mg/L. If levels are >1mg/L then the dosing interval is normally increased by 12 hours. 1 hour post dose (peak) levels may be measured aiming for a target of >20mg/L. If there is no change in the dosage regimen or renal function repeat peak levels every 3–4 days.

NOTES

- **Administration: IV:** slow IV injection over 3-5 minutes injected neat or diluted in NaCl 0.9% or glucose 5%. IV infusion over 30-60 minutes for high dose 'child – single daily dose regimen in an appropriate volume of fluid. Physically compatible with NaCl 0.9%, glucose 5% and 10%. Should not be mixed with penicillins, cephalosporins, erythromycin, heparin, sodium bicarbonate. Adequate flushing, or administration at separate sites, is suggested.

- Increased risk of ototoxicity and nephrotoxicity with cephalosporins, vancomycin, ciclosporin, cisplatin, diuretics such as furosemide, amphotericin.

Nifedipine

- **Tablets (modified release):** 10mg, 20mg, 40mg.
- **Tablets (slow release):** 30mg, 60mg.
- **Capsules:** 5mg, 10mg.
- **Capsules (modified release):** 10mg, 20mg.
- **Capsules (slow release):** 30mg.
- **Oral liquid:** 2% (20mg in 1mL, 1mg per 0.05mL drop).

DOSAGE

Route	Age				Frequency	Notes
	birth–1 month	1 month–2 years	2–12 years	12–18 years	(times daily)	
Oral	–	← 250–500 microgram/kg →			single dose	<u>Hypertensive crisis/angina.</u> Bite the capsules releasing the contents into the mouth and then swallow.

DOSAGE continued

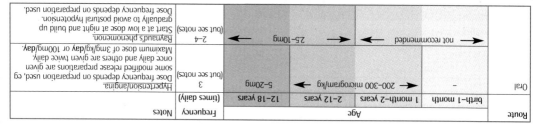

Route	Age				Frequency (times daily)	Notes
	birth–1 month	1 month–2 years	2–12 years	12–18 years		
Oral	–	← 200–300 microgram/kg →		5–20mg	3	Hypertension/angina. Dose frequency depends on preparation used, eg some modified release preparations are given once daily and others are given twice daily. Maximum dose of 3mg/kg/day or 100mg/day.
	← not recommended →		← 2.5–10mg →		2–4 (but see notes)	Raynaud's phenomenon. Start at a low dose at night and build up gradually to avoid postural hypotension. Dose frequency depends on preparation used.

NOTES

■ **Administration: oral:** if liquid preparation required for young children (and oral drops are not available), liquid can be aspirated from capsules. However different brands of nifedipine capsules contain different amounts of liquid: IVAX capsules contain 10mg nifedipine in 0.45mL; Bayer and APS capsules contain 10mg nifedipine in 0.3mL; Alphapharma capsules contain 10mg in 0.36mL; Hillcross capsules contain 10mg in 0.28mL. Aspirated liquid dose should be covered in foil and administered immediately as

■ Use the lower stated dose in hepatic impairment and monitor carefully.

■ May increase digoxin concentration.

■ Oral drops are available on a named patient basis via IDIS World Medicines.

■ Nifedipine should be prescribed by generic name, form and trade name as all products are not equivalent; see *Medicines for children* or *British National Formulary (BNF)* for details of trade names.

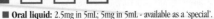

■ **Tablets:** 5mg.

■ **Oral liquid:** 2.5mg in 5mL; 5mg in 5mL - available as a 'special'.

DOSAGE

Route	Age				Frequency (times daily)	Notes
	birth–1 month	1 month–2 years	2–12 years	12–18 years		
Oral (epilepsy)	← 125 microgram/kg →			–	2	Usual starting dose.
	← 250 microgram/kg (maximum 500 microgram/kg) →			–	2	Usual target maintenance dose. Total daily dose may be divided into 3.

NOTES

■ Target maintenance dose should be reached over 2-3 weeks.

■ 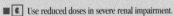 Use reduced doses in severe renal impairment.

■ Caution in severe liver disease; may precipitate coma.

■ Epilepsy is not a licensed indication in any age group. The 5mg in 5mL oral liquid is available as a 'special' from Rosemont and as such is unlicensed.

■ **Tablets:** 50mg, 100mg.
■ **Capsules:** 50mg, 100mg.

■ **Capsules (modified release):** 100mg.
■ **Suspension:** 25mg in 5mL.

DOSAGE

Route	Age				Frequency	Notes
	birth–1 month	1 month–2 years	2–12 years	12–18 years	(times daily)	
Oral	contra-indicated	≤3 months contra-indicated	750 microgram/kg	50–100mg	4	Treatment
		≥3 months 750 microgram/kg			4	
	–	–	–	100mg	2	Treatment (modified release capsule)
	contra-indicated	≤3 months contra-indicated	1mg/kg	50–100mg	1 (at night)	Prophylaxis
		≥3 months 1mg/kg			1 (at night)	

NOTES

■ **Administration: oral:** take with food or milk to minimise gastrointestinal reactions. The modified release capsules should be swallowed whole.

■ Although only small amounts appear in breast milk, these may be sufficient to produce haemolysis in G6PD-deficient infants and therefore nitrofurantoin should not be given to breast-feeding mothers.

- Nitrofurantoin should not be given to infants under 3 months of age or to pregnant patients at term (during labour and delivery) because of the theoretical possibility of haemolytic anaemia in the fetus or newborn infant due to immature erythrocyte enzyme systems.

- Tablets and capsules are licensed for use ≥3 months of age. The modified release capsules are licensed for use ≥12 years of age. The suspension is not licensed for use in the UK; it may be imported via IDIS.

Nystatin

- **Tablets:** 500,000 units.
- **Pastilles:** 100,000 units.

- **Oral suspension:** 100,000 units in 1mL.

DOSAGE

Newborn infant

Route	Age	Frequency	Notes
	birth–1 month	(times daily)	
Oral	1 mL	3	Prophylaxis administered after feeds.
	1 mL	4	Treatment administered after feeds.

L

Child

Route	Age			Frequency (times daily)	Notes
	1 month–2 years	2–12 years	12–18 years		
Oral	1mL	← 1mL or 1 pastille →		4	Intestinal or oral candidiasis.
	1mL	← 1mL or 1 pastille →		4 to 6	Oral candidiasis in the immunocompromised.
	5mL	← 5mL or 1 tablet →		4 to 6	Oesophageal/intestinal candidiasis in the immunocompromised.

Continue for 48 hours after clinical cure to prevent relapse.

NOTES

■ **Administration: oral:** in infants and children drop suspension into the mouth. In older children retain for 1 minute before swallowing. Pastilles are dissolved in the mouth. Administer after meal or feed.

■ Some nystatin suspensions contain sucrose.

Omeprazole

■ **Capsules:** 10mg, 20mg, 40mg.
■ **Tablets (dispersible):** 10mg, 20mg and 40 mg.

■ **Injection:** 40mg vial + 10mL solvent.
■ **Infusion:** 40mg.

DOSAGE

Route	Age			Frequency (times daily)	Notes
	1 month–2 years	2–12 years	12–18 years		
Oral	initially ← 700 microgram/kg → increasing as necessary to 3mg/kg/day		20–40mg	1	Dose should preferably be rounded to the nearest oral dose form. Initial dose is given once daily; higher doses may be given in 2 divided doses.
Oral for *H. pylori*	≥1 year ← 1–2mg/kg → rounded to nearest 10mg to a maximum of 40mg		40mg	1	Treatment for 14 days with amoxicillin and clarithromycin, or amoxicillin and metronidazole, or clarithromycin and metronidazole (see individual drug monographs for doses).
IV infusion/ IV injection	initially ← 500 microgram/kg → increasing as necessary to 2mg/kg/day		40mg	1	*There is limited data on IV administration in children. Initial dose is given once daily; higher doses may be given in 2 divided doses if necessary.

*The IV dose given above is based on the relative bioavailability by the oral and IV routes. There is very limited published information on IV doses in children.

NOTES

■ **Administration: oral:** if capsules cannot be swallowed whole then they can be opened and the intact enteric coated granules mixed in an acidic drink e.g. orange or apple juice and then swallowed without chewing.

Alternatively the MUPS® tablets can be dispersed in water, fruit juice or yogurt. For narrow bore nasogastric or PEG tubes the MUPS® tablets should be dispersed in a large volume of water or a suspension can be made using the granules in the capsules as follows: add the enteric-coated granules to 10mL of sodium bicarbonate 8.4% and leave to stand for about 10 minutes until a turbid suspension is formed. Administer the suspension immediately and flush the tube with water. The patient may be pre-treated with a solution of sodium bicarbonate 8.4%, to buffer the pH of the stomach. This is not necessary for administration via a jejunostomy tube as the jejunostomy pH is already alkaline. **Injection:** slow IV bolus over at least 2.5-5 minutes at a rate not exceeding 2mL per minute. The IV solution should be used within 4 hours of reconstitution. **Infusion:** the vial of omeprazole powder should be dissolved in 100mL of NaCl 0.9% or glucose 5% for infusion. No other solutions should be used. The infusion should then be given at a suitable rate. The infusion should be complete within 12 hours of reconstitution if NaCl 0.9% is used and within 3 hours if glucose is used. **NB.** Preparations for infusion and injection are distinct and separate.

■ Caution should be exercised in patients with hepatic impairment since both the bioavailability and the half-life of omeprazole may increase.

■ Oral preparations are licensed for use in children ≥2 years of age for the treatment of severe ulcerating reflux oesophagitis (treatment should be initiated by a hospital-based paediatrician). The injection and infusion are not licensed for use in children.

Ondansetron

■ **Tablets:** 4mg, 8mg.
■ **Tablets (melt formulation):** 4mg, 8mg.

■ **Oral solution:** 4mg in 5mL.
■ **Injection:** 2mg in 1mL; 2mL and 4mL ampoules.

DOSAGE

Indication	Route	Age			Frequency	Notes
		1 month-2 years	2-12 years	12-18 years	(times daily)	
Emetogenic chemotherapy	IV	← 5mg/m² → (maximum 8mg)		8mg	single dose (immediately prior to chemotherapy)	Can be repeated every 8-12 hours during chemotherapy and for at least 24 hours after treatment
		then				or
	Oral	← 4mg →		8mg	2	Give orally after initial IV dose. Continue oral treatment for up to 5 days after a course of treatment.
Postoperative nausea and vomiting (PONV)	IV slow injection	–	100 microgram/kg (maximum 4mg)	4mg	single dose	For prevention >12 years give at induction of anaesthesia; 2-12 years give prior to or after induction of anaesthesia. The same dose can be used for treatment of established PONV.

NOTES

■ **Administration: oral:** the melt tablets dissolve in mouth but they must be swallowed (not bucally absorbed). **IV:** bolus over 2-5 minutes; infusion over 15 minutes diluted in glucose 5% or NaCl 0.9%.

■ 🔲 In patients with marked hepatic impairment, clearance is significantly reduced.

Dioralyte® sachets, **Dioralyte®** relief sachets, **Dioralyte®** effervescent tablets.
Diocalm Junior® sachets; **Rehidrat®** sachets; **Electrolade®** sachets.
(see *Medicines for Children* for full product details).

DOSAGE/ADMINISTRATION
According to fluid loss:
Infant: 1–1½ × usual 24 hour feed volume or 150 mL/kg/day given in divided doses.
Child: 200mL solution after each loose motion.
Adult: 200-400mL solution after each loose motion.
Powder in sachets: reconstitute the sachets with the quantity of water recommended i.e. 250mL for Rehidrat®, 200mLs for other preparations. Use sterile or freshly boiled and cooled water for infants.
Effervescent tablets: dissolve 2 tablets in 200mL of water. Only use for adults and children ≥1 year of age.

NOTES

■ All the preparations are licensed for use in all ages with the exception of Dioralyte® effervescent tablets which are not licensed for use <1 year of age.

■ **Tablets:** 2.5mg, 3mg, 5mg.
■ **Oral liquid:** 2.5mg in 5mL; 5mg in 5mL.

■ **Intravesical instillation:** 5mg in 30 mL.

DOSAGE

Route	Age			Frequency (times daily)	Notes
	2–12 years		12–18 years		
Oral	<5 years 1.25–2.5mg	>5 years 2.5–5mg	5mg	2–3	12–18 years - maximum dose of 5mg four times daily.
Intravesical instillation	5mg		5mg	2–3	

NOTES

■ [L] Licensed for use >5 years of age for nocturnal enuresis and neurogenic bladder disorders. The intravesical preparation and the 5mg in 5mL elixir are unlicensed products.

■ The 5mg in 5mL oral liquid is available as a 'special' from Rosemont. The intravesical preparation is available on a named patient basis from Sanofi-Synthelabo.

Injection: 2mg in 1mL; 2mL ampoule.

DOSAGE

Newborn infant

Route	Age	Frequency	Notes
	birth–1 month	(times daily)	
IV loading	100 microgram/kg	single dose	
IV maintenance	50 microgram/kg	4–6	As need arises.

Child

Route	Age			Frequency	Notes
	1 month–2 years	2–12 years	12–18 years	(times daily)	
IV	← 60–100 microgram/kg →			single dose	Initial dose. Subsequent doses 10-20microgram/kg– adjust dose and interval as required.

NOTES

- **Administration: IV: bolus** – administer neat or diluted in NaCl 0.9% or glucose 5%.

- Use with caution in severe renal impairment as duration of action is prolonged.

- **Tablets**: 500mg.
- **Tablets (dispersible)**: 120mg, 500mg.
- **Oral solution/suspension**: 120mg in 5mL, 250mg in 5mL.
- **Suppositories**: 30mg, 60mg, 120mg, 125mg, 240mg, 250mg, 500mg, 1g.

DOSAGE

Analgesic/antipyretic/post-operative pain relief – Newborn infant

Route	Age			Frequency (times daily)	Notes
	Pre-term 28-32 weeks	Pre-term 32-36 weeks	birth-1 month		
Oral loading dose	←	20mg/kg	→	single dose	
Oral maintenance dose	15mg/kg	-		12 hourly	Maximum **daily** dose 30mg/kg.
	-	← 20mg/kg	→	8 hourly	Maximum **daily** dose 60mg/kg.
Rectal loading dose	20mg/kg	← 30mg/kg	→	single dose	
Rectal maintenance dose	15mg/kg	-		12 hourly	Maximum **daily** dose 30mg/kg.
	-	← 20mg/kg	→	8 hourly	Maximum **daily** dose 60mg/kg.

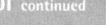

Child – analgesic/antipyretic

Route	Age			Frequency	Notes
	1 month-2 years	2-12 years	12-18 years	(times daily)	
Oral loading dose	← 20mg/kg →		-	single dose	
Oral maintenance dose	1-3 months 20mg/kg			8 hourly	Maximum **total dose in 24 hours:** <3 months: 60mg/kg
	> 3 months ← 15mg/kg →		500mg - 1g	4-6 hourly	>3 months - 12 years: 90mg/kg >12 years: 4g.
Rectal loading dose	1-3 months 30mg/kg		-	single dose	
	> 3 months ← 40mg/kg →				
Rectal maintenance dose	← 20mg/kg →		500mg - 1g	1-3 months 8 hourly > 3 months 4-6 hourly	Maximum **total dose in 24 hours:** <3 months: 60mg/kg >3 months - 12 years: 90mg/kg >12 years: 4g.

Post-operative pain relief (over 3 months)

The total daily dose may be increased to 90mg/kg/day (maximum 4g) orally or rectally, for 48 hours. Give loading dose of 20mg/kg then 15mg/kg orally or 30mg/kg then 20mg/kg rectally up to 4 hourly. Give regular doses for first 24–48 hours.

NOTES

■ 🔲 Licensed >2 months of age for post immunisation pyrexia and >3 months of age as an antipyretic and analgesic. The 30mg and 1g suppositories are available as 'specials' from several hospital manufacturing units and as such are unlicensed.

■ 🄲 Not significantly removed by CAPD.

■ See *Medicines for Children* for details of treatment of paracetamol poisoning.

■ 🄲 In moderate impairment (creatinine clearance 10-50mL/min/1.73m^2) dose interval not less than 6 hours; in severe impairment (creatinine clearance <10mL/min/1.73m^2) dose interval not less than 8 hours. Significantly removed by haemodialysis; give dose after haemodialysis.

■ 🄿 Liver failure: dose related toxicity. Avoid large doses.

■ **Injection:** 5mL and 10mL ampoules.

■ **Enema:** equal parts paraldehyde and olive oil, arachis oil or sunflower oil.

DOSAGE

Status epilepticus

Route		Age			Frequency	Notes
	birth–1 month	1 month–2 years	2–12 years	12–18 years		
Rectal	→	0.4mL/kg	←	5–10mL	single dose	Doses stated in mL/kg or as mL of paraldehyde. Dilute with an equal volume of olive, arachis or sunflower oil before administration, or if using a ready-prepared 'special', remember that it is already diluted and dose accordingly.

NOTES

■ **Administration: rectal:** enema is extemporaneously prepared immediately prior to use using equal parts paraldehyde and olive oil or sunflower oil; avoid using arachis oil to dilute the enema in peanut allergy. A plastic syringe may be used to measure paraldehyde if the contact time is less than 10 minutes; if not use a glass syringe.

■ The enema is prepared extemporaneously or available as a 'special' from Martindale Pharmaceuticals Ltd and as such is unlicensed.

■ Tablets: 50mg.

■ Injection: 50mg in 1mL, 1mL & 2mL ampoules; 10mg in 1mL, 5mL & 10mL ampoules.

DOSAGE

Route	Age				Frequency (times daily)	Notes
	birth–1 month	1 month–2 years	2–12 years	12–18 years		
Oral	500 microgram –1mg/kg	◄— 500 microgram/kg–2mg/kg —►		50–100mg	single dose	< 2 months: can be repeated every 10-12 hours.
SC/IM	500 microgram –1mg/kg	◄— 500 microgram/kg–2mg/kg —►		25–100mg	single dose	≥2 months: can be repeated every 4-6 hours. Neonates and infants <1 year show an increased susceptibility to respiratory depression.
IV bolus	◄— 500 microgram/kg–1mg/kg —►			25– 50mg	single dose	
IV infusion	–	◄— 1mg/kg then 100–400 microgram/kg/hour —►			loading dose; continuous infusion	Ventilated patients may require higher doses. Adjust according to response.

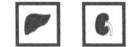

NOTES

■ **Administration: IV:** for IV infusion dilute with NaCl 0.9% or glucose 5% to required volume. Solutions are physically stable for at least 24 hours. For IV bolus dilute to 10mg per mL with Water for Injections and give over 2-5 minutes.

■ Avoid in acute respiratory depression and paralytic ileus.

■ Use with caution in raised intra-cranial pressure and head injury.

■ 📋 Avoid in liver disease – may precipitate coma.

■ 🄲 Avoid in severe renal impairment.

Phenobarbital (phenobarbitone) (controlled drug)

■ **Tablets:** 15 mg, 30 mg, 60 mg.
■ **Oral liquid:** 50mg in 5mL ('special' or extemporaneously prepared; various strengths can be prepared).

■ **Elixir:** 15mg in 5mL; contains alcohol and is not recommended.
■ **Injection:** 200mg in 1mL; other strengths are available as 'specials'.

DOSAGE

Route	Age				Frequency (times daily)	Notes
	birth–1 month	1 month–2 years	2–12 years	12–18 years		
Oral	Give an IV loading dose	← 1–1.5mg/kg →		60–180mg	2	<u>Antiepileptic.</u> Starting dose.

DOSAGE continued

Route	Age				Frequency (times daily)	Notes
	birth– 1 month	1 month– 2 years	2–12 years	12–18 years		
Oral	2.5–5mg/kg	← 2.5–4mg/kg →		–	2*	<u>Antiepileptic.</u> Usual target maintenance dose.
	–	–		60–180mg	1	
IV slow bolus	←	20mg/kg then 2.5–5mg/kg	→	20mg/kg then 300mg/dose	single dose then 2*	<u>Status epilepticus</u> loading dose then . maintenance

* The plasma half-life is long in the neonatal period (2–4 days) and therefore once daily dosing is adequate but it decreases with age and is halved after 1–2 weeks of medication because the drug acts to induce liver enzymes.

NOTES

■ **Administration: IV:** the 200mg in 1mL injection should be diluted 1 in 10 with Water for Injections; other injection strengths should also be adequately diluted e.g. 30mg in 1mL ampoules are often diluted with an equal quantity of Water for Injections (giving a solution of 15mg in 1mL) and used in neonates. Give no faster than 1 mg/kg/minute. Avoid umbilical artery cannula injection in neonates.

■ Ⓒ ☞ Monitor levels in renal and liver disease and adjust dosage as necessary; usual target concentration is a trough level at 7-14 days of 10-25mg/L.

Phenobarbital (phenobarbitone) (controlled drug) continued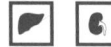

- Enzyme-inducer which interacts with other drugs including other anti-convulsants.

- Phenobarbital is a controlled drug which must fulfil controlled drug prescription requirements except for the own handwriting requirement.

- The 200 mg in 1mL injection and the tablets are licensed for use in children and adults; other preparations are available as 'specials' or can be extemporaneously prepared and are therefore unlicensed.

Phenoxymethylpenicillin (penicillin V)

- **Tablets:** 250mg.

- **Oral solution:** 125mg in 5mL, 250mg in 5mL.

DOSAGE

Route	Age			Frequency (times daily)	Notes
	1 month–2 years	2–12 years	12–18 years		
Oral	≤1 year 62.5mg	2–5 years 125mg	500mg (750mg in severe infection)	4	Treatment doses.
	1–2 years 125mg	6–12 years 250mg		4	

Route	Age			Frequency (times daily)	Notes
	1 month–2 years	2–12 years	12–18 years		
Oral	<u><1 year</u> 62.5mg	<u>2–5 years</u> 125mg	500mg	2	Pneumococcal infection prophylaxis.
	<u>1–2 years</u> 125mg	<u>6–12 years</u> 250mg		2	
	←	250mg	→	2	Rheumatic fever prophylaxis.

NOTES

- **Administration: oral:** take an hour before food or on an empty stomach or 2 hours after food.

- Contra-indicated in penicillin hypersensitivity.

Phenytoin

- **Tablets:** phenytoin sodium 50mg, 100mg.
- **Tablets (chewable):** phenytoin base 50mg.
- **Capsules:** phenytoin sodium 25mg, 50mg, 100mg, 300mg.

- **Oral liquid:** phenytoin base 30mg in 5mL, 90mg in 5mL.
- **Injection:** phenytoin sodium 50mg in 1mL, 5mL ampoule.

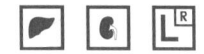

DOSAGE

Indication	Route	Age				Frequency	Notes
		birth – 1 month	1 month – 2 years	2 – 12 years	12 – 18 years	(times daily)	
Antiepileptic	Oral	Use IV loading dose.	← 1.5–2.5mg/kg →		75–150mg	2	Starting dose.
		2–4mg/kg	← 2.5–5mg/kg →		150–200mg	2	Usual target maintenance dose.
		7.5mg/kg	← 7.5mg/kg →		300mg	2	Usual maximum dose.
	IV	20mg/kg	← 18mg/kg →			single dose	Loading dose (over 30–45 minutes).
		← 2.5–5mg/kg →			–	2	Usual maintenance dose (over 30 minutes).
		–	–	–	100mg	3–4	
Anti – arrhythmic	IV	–	← 18mg/kg →			single dose	

NOTES

■ **Administration: oral:** bioavailability of oral phenytoin may be reduced by enteral and/or nasogastric tube feeds and may be erratic in neonates, otherwise oral bioavailability is similar to IV. Note: different preparations contain different forms of phenytoin base or phenytoin sodium. **IV:** IV injection must be given slowly at approximately 1 mg/kg/minute to avoid hypotension and/or arrhythmias. Monitor blood pressure and ECG. May be diluted in NaCl 0.9% injection ONLY, to a concentration not greater than 10mg in 1mL. This dilution may be filtered without loss of activity. An in-line filter (0.22-0.50microns) should be used. Avoid rapid flushing of IV lines which may deliver a bolus of phenytoin. Do not mix with glucose or other drugs because this can cause precipitation of phenytoin acid.

■ **Dose adjustment:** increase oral dose by no more than 1 mg/kg/day. Measure phenytoin blood level after 1 week and as required. Full intravenous dose only to be given if patient not on phenytoin or if blood level less than 2.5 mg/L. If blood level is 10-20 mg/L 2 hours after loading dose completed, start maintenance dose 12 hours after loading dose complete. If blood level is less than 10 mg/L 2 hours after loading dose is completed, give a further loading dose of 5 mg/kg over 20 minutes at once and commence maintenance dose after 8 hours.

■ 100mg phenytoin sodium is equivalent to 90mg phenytoin base.

■ Reduce dose in liver disease. In renal disease dose adjustment may be required.

■ Preparations licensed for use in the appropriate ages with the exception of the 90mg/5mL oral liquid which is available as a 'special' from Rosemont.

■ **Injection:** 2.25g (2g piperacillin with 0.25g tazobactam) and 4.5g (4g piperacillin with 0.5g tazobactam).

DOSAGE

Newborn infant (birth to 1 month)

Route	Age	Frequency	Notes
	birth–1month	(times daily)	
IV	90mg/kg	3	

Child

Route	Age			Frequency	Notes
	1 month–2 years	2–12 years	12–18 years	(times daily)	
IV	←	90mg/kg	→	4	Maximum single dose is 4.5g.

Dose adjustment in renal impairment

Creatinine clearance (mL/minute/1.73m²)	Dose	Frequency (times daily)
40–80	90mg/kg (maximum 4.5g)	4
20–40	90mg/kg (maximum 4.5g)	3

NOTES

■ **Administration:** on reconstitution 1g displaces 0.7mL. **IV:** for IV bolus, reconstitute to 200mg in 1mL and give over 3-5 minutes; for IV infusion dilute to 80mg in 1mL and give over 20-40 minutes. **IM:** not recommended for use in children. Do not mix with aminoglycosides; do not administer through the same line without adequate flushing in-between.

■ Contra-indicated in penicillin hypersensitivity.

■ Reduce dose in moderate renal impairment (see table). In haemodialysis ensure dose is given post dialysis, and give 45mg/kg three times daily.

■ Licensed for use in all ages, but only licensed <12 years for sepsis in neutropenia and licensed for appendicitis complicated by rupture with peritonitis and/or abscess formation in children aged 2-12 years. The doses quoted reflect use in severe sepsis in neutropenia.

Potassium chloride

■ **Tablets (slow release):** 600mg (8mmol K$^+$).
■ **Tablets (effervescent):** 6.7mmol each of K$^+$ and Cl$^-$; 12mmol K$^+$ and 8mmol Cl$^-$.
■ **Liquid:** 1mmol in 1mL of K$^+$ and Cl$^-$.

■ **Injection:** 15% (2mmol in 1mL K$^+$ and Cl$^-$).
■ **IV fluid:** with added potassium – see IV fluids guidance section in *Medicines for Children*.

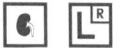

DOSAGE

Indication	Route	Age			Frequency (times daily)	Notes
		1 month–2 years	2–12 years	12–18 years		
Potassium supplement	Oral/IV	←	0.5–1mmol/kg	→	2	IV administration should be in a suitable infusion fluid or as part of a suitable intravenous feeding regimen.
Acute hypokalaemia	IV infusion	←	0.08–0.2mmol/kg/hour	→	continuous	Always check the dose carefully, an overdose can be rapidly fatal. Recheck the potassium level after 3 hours.

NOTES

■ **Administration: oral:** take with or after food. Total daily dose can be given in three or more divided doses to minimise gastric irritation. **IV:** use premixed bags in preference whenever practicable. Dilute injection before use with not less than 50 times its volume of IV fluids and mix well. Usual maximum concentration for infusion is 40mmol K$^+$/L given at a rate not exceeding 0.2mmol/kg/hour. Higher concentrations and rates require ECG

and electrolyte monitoring. **Extreme care should be exercised when calculating infusion doses.**

■ Avoid routine use in renal impairment; high risk of hyperkalaemia. Monitor plasma potassium levels and review regularly.

■ Slow release tablets are not licensed for use in children; other preparations are licensed for use in both adults and children.

■ The National Patient Safety Agency (NPSA) alert re: potassium chloride concentrate solutions (see www.npsa.org.uk for further details), includes the following advice:

1. Potassium chloride concentrate solutions are restricted to critical care areas only and should be stored in a separate locked cupboard. Documentation should follow the pattern for controlled drugs and the concentrate should not be transferred between clinical areas.

2. Commercially prepared, ready to use, diluted solutions should be prescribed and used wherever possible.

3. A second practitioner check is required for any IV solution prepared from the concentrate.

Prednisolone

■ **Tablets:** 1mg, 5mg, 25mg.
■ **Tablets (dispersible):** 5mg.
■ **Tablets (enteric coated):** 2.5mg, 5mg.
■ **Injection:** 25mg in 1mL.

■ **Suppositories:** 5mg.
■ **Retention enema:** 20mg in 100mL.
■ **Rectal foam:** 20mg per metered actuation.

DOSAGE

Indication	Route	Age			Frequency (times daily)	Notes
		1 month–2 years	2–12 years	12–18 years		
Acute asthma	Oral	← 1–2mg/kg (maximum dose 40mg) →			1	Treat for 1–5 days and then stop; no need to taper dose.
Suppression of inflammatory and allergic disorders	Oral	← 1–2mg/kg →			1	The daily dose can be given in 2–3 divided doses if necessary. Consider alternate day treatment in long term.
Croup requiring intubation	Oral	← 1mg/kg →		–	2	Start within 24 hours of intubation continuing until 24 hours after extubation.
Nephrotic syndrome	Oral	← 60mg/m² (maximum dose 80mg) → then			1 (morning)	Initial dose (on presentation) for 4 weeks. Then (providing proteinuria has been absent for 3 days) maintenance. Maintenance dose for 4 weeks then stop. Repeat course for any relapses.
		← 40mg/m² (maximum dose 60mg) →			1 (alternate days)	
Replacement	Oral	–		2.5mg/m²	2	In some cases, could be used as a 5mg/m² once daily dose.
Autoimmune hepatitis	Oral	← 2mg/kg (maximum dose 40mg) →			1	

Indication	Route	Age			Frequency	Notes
		1 month–2 years	2–12 years	12–18 years	(times daily)	
Inflammatory bowel disease	Oral	–	← 1–2mg/kg → (maximum 60mg daily)		1	Give as a reducing regimen, aiming to 'wean off' over a few weeks if possible.
JIA, connective tissue disease, vasculitis	Oral	← up to 2mg/kg →			1 (morning or on alternate days)	Use the lowest dose that controls the disease without unacceptable side-effects.
	IM	← dose must be individualised →			single dose	Dose depends on the condition being treated and its severity.
Local treatment of ulcerative colitis and Crohn's disease	Rectal (enema)	–	–	1 enema	1	At bedtime for 2–4 weeks, continued if good response.
Proctitis and distal ulcerative colitis	Rectal (foam)	–	–	1 metered dose	1–2	For 2 weeks, continued for a further 2 weeks if good response.

DOSAGE continued

Indication	Route	Age			Frequency (times daily)	Notes
		1 month–2 years	2–12 years	12–18 years		
Proctitis and rectal complications of Crohn's disease	Rectal (suppository)	–	← 1 suppository →		2	Night and morning after bowel movement.
Infantile spasms; epileptic seizures	Oral	← 2mg/kg →			1	Higher doses have been used in infantile spasms.

NOTES

■ **Administration: oral:** the uncoated tablets are scored and can be halved, and these and the dispersible tablets should be taken with or after food in order to minimise gastrointestinal side effects. The enteric coated tablets should be swallowed whole, but must not be used in cystic fibrosis.

■ Use is contra-indicated in patients with systemic infection, unless specific anti-infective therapy is used.

■ Live vaccines should not be given to patients receiving immunosuppressive doses of steroids.

■ **Withdrawal of corticosteroids:** in patients who have received systemic corticosteroids for greater than 3 weeks, withdrawal should not be abrupt. However, abrupt withdrawal is appropriate in some patients treated for up to 3 weeks if it is considered that the disease is unlikely to relapse or that the dose has been such that abrupt withdrawal is unlikely to lead to clinically relevant hypothalamic-pituitary-adrenal suppression.

■ The retention enema and rectal foam are not licensed for use in children.

■ **Tablets:** 10mg, 25mg.
■ **Oral liquid:** 5mg in 5mL.

■ **Injection:** 25mg in 1mL (2.5%); 1mL and 2mL ampoules.

DOSAGE

Indication	Route	Age			Frequency	Notes
		1 month–2 years	2–12 years	12–18 years	(times daily)	
Symptomatic relief of allergy	Oral	<u>≤1 year</u> 2.5–5mg <u>>1 year</u> 5–10mg	<u>≤6 years</u> 5–10mg <u>>6 years</u> 10–15mg	10–20mg	2–3 2–3	When 3 doses in 24 hours are given, use the lower stated amount.
Sedation	Oral	**DOSE BY WEIGHT** ← 1–2mg/kg →		–	single dose	Give at bedtime for night sedation. For daytime sedation give once, or twice daily using the lower dose.
		DOSE BY AGE <u>≤1 year</u> 5–10mg <u>>1 year</u> 10–20mg	<u>2–5 years</u> 10–20mg <u>6–10 years</u> 20–25mg <u>>10 years</u> 25–50mg	25–50mg	single dose single dose single dose	
Sedation on intensive care units	IV slow bolus/oral/ deep IM	500 microgram – 1mg/kg (maximum 25mg)		25–50mg	4	Start at low dose and adjust according to response. May be used in conjunction with chloral hydrate (up to 50mg/kg).

NOTES

■ **Administration: IV:** for slow IV injection dilute the 2.5% solution to 10 times its volume with Water for Injections immediately prior to use and give over at least 5 minutes.

■ Contra-indicated in neonates, premature infants, porphyria, patients in coma or suffering CNS depression of any cause. Caution in use <1 year of age because of a possible association with sudden infant death syndrome.

■ L E Licensed for use ≥2 years of age.

Propofol

L R

■ **Injection:** 10mg in 1mL (1%); 20mL ampoule, 50mL and 100mL bottles, 50mL vial, 50mL pre-filled syringe. 20mg in 1mL (2%), 50ml vial, prefilled syringe.

DOSAGE

Newborn infant – not recommended

Child

Indication	Route	Age			Frequency	Notes
		1 month–2 years	2–12 years	12–18 years	(times daily)	
Induction of general anaesthesia	IV bolus	← 2.5mg/kg →		1.5–2.5mg/kg	single dose	Adjust dose according to response. Large doses are often required for children under 8 years of age. Lower doses recommended for children of ASA grades 3 and 4.

Indication	Route	Age			Frequency	Notes
		1 month–2 years	2–12 years	12–18 years	(times daily)	
Maintenance of general anaesthesia	IV infusion	9–15mg/kg/hour with Propofol-Lipuro 1%	<3 years see 1 month–2 years ≥3 years 9–15mg/kg/hour	4–12mg/kg/hour	continuous continuous	Only the Propofol-Lipuro 1% is licensed for >1 month-3 years of age for maintenance of general anaesthesia. Adjust dose according to response.

NOTES

■ Do not use for sedation in intensive care.

■ **Administration: IV**: inject slowly or infuse undiluted. If required, propofol may be diluted in glucose 5% only. Dilutions must not exceed 2mg in 1mL. Administer diluted solutions using PVC giving sets. Discard any diluted solution after 6 hours.

■ 🔲 Licensed for the induction of anaesthesia ≥1 month of age and maintenance of anaesthesia ≥3 years of age, with the exception of the brand of 1% Propofol-Lipuro® which is licenced >1 month. Not licensed for sedation in children.

260 Propranolol

L R

■ **Tablets:** 10mg, 40mg, 80mg, 160mg.
■ **Capsules (slow-release):** 80mg, 160mg.

■ **Oral solution:** 5mg in 5mL, 10mg in 5mL, 50mg in 5mL.
■ **Injection:** 1mg in 1mL.

DOSAGE

Indication	Route	Age				Frequency (times daily)	Notes
		birth – 1 month	1 month – 2 years	2 – 12 years	12 – 18 years		
Dysrhythmias	Oral	← 250-500 microgram/kg →			10-40mg	3-4	
	IV bolus	← 25-50 microgram/kg →			1mg	single dose	Repeat as necessary up to 4 times daily. Adults may receive repeated doses up to 10mg in total. Give slowly (over 5 minutes) under ECG control.
Tetralogy of Fallot	Oral	← 250 microgram/kg-1mg/kg →				2 (neonate) 3-4 (>1month)	
	IV bolus	← up to 100 microgram/kg →				single dose	Give slowly (over 5 minutes) under ECG control and repeat as necessary; 2 times daily in a neonate; 4 times daily in child <1 month of age.
Hypertrophic obstructive cardio-myopathy	Oral	← 250-500 microgram/kg →			10-40mg	3-4	This dose may be increased up to 2mg/kg four times daily with monitoring of heart rate and serum level.

DOSAGE continued

Indication	Route	Age				Frequency (times daily)	Notes
		birth – 1 month	1 month – 2 years	2 – 12 years	12 – 18 years		
Hypertension	Oral	250–500 microgram/kg	← 250 microgram/kg –1mg/kg →		–	3	Increase if necessary to a maximum of 2mg/kg/dose in neonates. In children, increase at weekly intervals as required, usual dose is 1–5mg/kg/day.
		–	–	–	80–160mg	2	
Hyper-thyroidism, including neonatal thyrotoxicosis.	Oral	←	250–750 microgram/kg	→		3	Increase dose according to response. May need up tp 1mg/kg three times a day.
Migraine prophylaxis	Oral	–	–	20mg	20–40mg	2–3	Licensed in all ages but evidence for efficacy at licensed doses is >6 years. Lower doses used in comparative trial which included children of 3 years.
Essential tremour	Oral	–	–	20mg	20–40mg	2–3	

NOTES

■ **Administration: IV:** give by slow IV bolus over at least 3-5 minutes. Compatible with glucose 5% and NaCl 0.9%. Incompatible with sodium bicarbonate.

■ The slow release capsules are not licensed for use in children.

■ See propanolol monograph in *Medicines for Children* for further information re: contra-indications, interactions, etc.

Pyridoxine

Tablets: 20mg, 50mg.
Oral liquid: 300mg in 5mL.

Injection: 50mg in 2mL.

DOSAGE

Indication	Route	Age				Frequency (times daily)	Notes
		birth – 1 month	1 month – 2 years	2 – 12 years	12 – 18 years		
Metabolic indications. Wilson's disease	Oral	←	50–250mg		→	1 or 2	Higher doses may help in partially responsive cases.

Indication	Route	Age				Frequency (times daily)	Notes
		birth – 1 month	1 month – 2 years	2 – 12 years	12 – 18 years		
Pyridoxine dependent seizures	Oral	50–100mg	-	-	-	1 or 2	<u>Test.</u> May be repeated on 2 more days.
		25–100mg	-	-	-	2	Usual maintenance dose.
		-	← 20–50mg →		-	1 or 2	Usual maintenance dose, but up to 500mg twice daily may be required
	IV bolus	50–100mg	← 25–100mg →		-	single dose	<u>Test.</u> May be repeated on 2 more days. If seizures cease, change to oral.
Prevention of isoniazid neuropathy	Oral	5mg	← 5–10mg →		10mg	1	Neurological side-effects of isoniazid are less common in children. Pyridoxine is given as prophylaxis if considered necessary; risk factors are malnutrition, diabetes, and chronic renal failure.

NOTES

■ **Administration: IV:** give over at least 5 minutes, dilute with NaCl 0.9%. Resuscitation facilities must be available when given IV. Monitor EEG while injecting.

■ Ⓛ Indications outlined in the table are unlicensed indications for pyridoxine. The injection and the oral liquid are available as 'specials' from Martindale, and as such are unlicensed.

■**Tablets:** 150mg, 300mg.
■**Tablets (effervescent):** 150mg, 300mg.

DOSAGE

■**Oral liquid:** 75mg in 5mL.
■**Injection:** 25mg in 1ml; 2mL ampoule.

Newborn infant

Route	Age	Frequency	Notes
	birth–1 month	(times daily)	
Oral/IV bolus	1mg/kg	3	Oral experience very limited in newborn infants.
IV infusion	30–60 microgram/kg/hour	continuous	Neonate in ITU – limited data. Maximum 3mg/kg/day.

Child

Route	Age			Frequency	Notes
	1 month-2 years	2-12 years	12-18 year	(times daily)	
Oral	≤6 months as for newborn infant ≥6 months as for 2-12 years	2-4mg/kg (maximum 150mg)	150mg	2	Doses of up to 9mg/kg/**day** have been used.
IV bolus	←	1mg/kg	→	2-4	Doses of up to 3mg/kg have been used - anecdotal. Standard adult dose is 50mg 3 times daily.

NOTES

- **Administration: oral:** the effervescent tablets should be completely dissolved in 75mL of water before swallowing; in cystic fibrosis, give 1-2 hours before food. **IV:** dilute to 2.5mg in 1mL with NaCl 0.9% or glucose 5% and give as a bolus over 3-5 minutes or further dilute and give as an infusion.

- Effervescent tablets contain aspartame and a high level of sodium.

- Reduce dose by approximately 50% in severe renal impairment.

- Oral treatment of peptic ulceration is the only licensed indication in children. The parenteral route is unlicensed for use in children.

Rifampicin

- **Capsules:** 150mg, 300mg.
- **Syrup:** 100mg in 5mL.
- **IV infusion:** 300mg, 600mg.

DOSAGE

Route	Age				Frequency (times daily)	Notes
	birth–1 month	1 month-2 years	2-12 years	12-18 years		
Oral or IV infusion over 2–3 hours	10mg/kg	← 10mg/kg → (maximum 600mg)		≤50 kg 450mg	1	Tuberculosis, in combination with other drugs. Treatment should always be given in collaboration with a specialist experienced in tuberculosis treatment.
				≥50 kg 600mg	1	

DOSAGE continued

Route	Age				Frequency (times daily)	Notes
	birth–1 month	1 month–2 years	2–12 years	12–18 years		
Oral	5mg/kg	<u><1 year</u> 5mg/kg <u>>1 year</u> 10mg/kg	← 10mg/kg → (maximum 600mg)		2 2	<u>Prophylaxis</u> in contacts of patients with meningococcal infection or elimination of nasal carriage. Administer for 2 days. <u>Treatment</u> of staphylococcal infection for 10-14 days.
	10mg/kg	<u><3 months</u> 10mg/kg <u>>3 months</u> 20mg/kg	← 20mg/kg → (maximum 600mg)		1 1	<u>Prophylaxis</u> in contacts of patients with invasive *Haemophilus influenzae* type B infection. Administer for 4 days.
IV infusion over 2-3 hours	–	← 20mg/kg → (maximum 600mg)			1	<u>Treatment</u> of tuberculous meningitis.
Oral	–	← 5–10mg/kg → (maximum dose 600mg)			1	Pruritus due to cholestasis.

Route	Age				Frequency (times daily)	Notes
	birth–1 month	1 month–2 years	2–12 years	12–18 years		
Oral for cystic fibrosis patients	-	←	10–20mg/kg	→	1	Reserved for MRSA infection or serious *S. aureus* infection that does not respond to other anti-staphylococcal drugs. Maximum dose of 1.2g.

NOTES

- **Administration: oral:** take oral preparations 30-60 minutes before or 2 hours after food. **IV:** infuse over 2-3 hours in glucose 5%, glucose 10% or NaCl 0.9% at a concentration of 1.2mg in 1mL. Discard after 6 hours.

- Avoid altogether in liver failure, or reduce antituberculosis and prophylaxis doses to 8mg/kg daily.

- Induces liver enzymes and reduces plasma levels of many drugs e.g. anticoagulants, ciclosporin, phenytoin, phenobarbital, theophylline, digoxin, most benzodiazepines, fluconazole. Dose adjustment of these may be necessary.

- When rifampicin is given during the last few weeks of pregnancy it may cause neonatal bleeding for which treatment with vitamin K_1 may be indicated.

- Rifampicin colours urine and other secretions red. Soft contact lenses may be permanently stained.

- Licensed for use in all ages, however, pruritis due to cholestasis is not a licensed indication.

- **Tablets:** 2mg, 4mg.
- **Tablets (modified release):** 4mg, 8mg.
- **Capsules (modified release):** 4mg, 8mg.
- **Oral solution:** 2mg in 5mL.
- **Aerosol inhaler/ CFC-free inhaler/ Breath-actuated inhaler:** 100 microgram per actuation.
- **Dry powder devices:** 200, 400 microgram per blister/capsule – Ventodisks® ; 200microgram per blister – Accuraler®.
- **Dry powder inhaler:** 95 microgram/actuation – Clickhaler®.
- **Nebuliser solution:** 2.5mg in 2.5mL; 5mg in 2.5mL – nebules; 5mg in 1mL-respirator solution.
- **Injection:** 500 microgram in 1mL, 1mL ampoule; 100 microgram in 1mL, 50mL vial.
- **Infusion:** 1mg in 1mL, 5mL ampoule.

DOSAGE

Route	Age				Frequency (times daily)	Notes
	birth–1 month	1 month–2 years	2–12 years	12–18 years		
Oral	–	100 microgram/kg	2-6 years 1mg 6-12 years 2mg	2-4mg	3-4 3-4	<u>Asthma:</u> reliever for symptom relief only.
Oral (modified release)	–	–	>3 years 4mg	8mg	2	
Aerosol inhaler	–	←	up to 1mg	→	single dose	<u>Asthma:</u> reliever, acute treatment given as required, 1-2 hourly initially then reduce

Route	Age				Frequency (times daily)	Notes
	birth-1 month	1 month-2 years	2-12 years	12-18 years		
Inhaled Ventodisks®	-	-	← ≥5 years → 200-400 micrograms		single dose	Asthma: reliever, on demand, routine use.
Inhaled Accuhaler®	-	-	← ≥5 years → 200 microgram		single dose	Asthma: reliever, on demand, routine use.
Nebuliser solution	1.25-2.5mg	← 2.5-5mg →			single dose	Asthma: reliever given as required.1-2 hourly initially then reduce frequency to 4-6 hourly in hospital with monitoring. In severe acute asthma half hourly doses may be given in hospital. NB. Only licensed for use up to 4 times daily.
IV bolus over 5 minutes	← 5 microgram/kg →		← 15 microgram/kg → (maximum 250 microgram)		single dose	Status asthmaticus
IV bolus	← 4 microgram/kg →				single dose	Renal hyperkalaemia:-repeat if necessary.
Nebuliser	← 2.5-5mg →				single dose	Renal hyperkalaemia:-repeat if necessary.

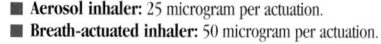

NOTES

■ **Administration: oral:** sustained release tablets and capsules should not be crushed or chewed. **Nebulisation:** nebules can be diluted with NaCl 0.9% or mixed with ipratropium or budesonide nebuliser solutions (NOT fluticasone). **Inhaled:** inhaler devices may be used with a Volumatic® spacer device; other spacers are available for use with salbutamol inhaler e.g. Aerochamber®. **IV:** IV bolus must be given over at least 5 minutes at a maximum concentration of 50 microgram in 1mL. The 500 microgram in 1mL strength should be diluted with Water for Injections. IV infusion should be diluted in glucose 5%, NaCl 0.9% or glucose 4%/NaCl 0.18%, although it may, if necessary, be given undiluted via a central line in intensive care. Note: some units are using 200 microgram in 1mL (peripherally) and others, 500 microgram in 1mL (centrally) in fluid restricted patients. IV solution is compatible with potassium; incompatible with aminophylline.

■ Modified release tablets and capsules are licensed for use ≥3 years of age. Oral solution is licensed for use ≥2 years of age. Injection not licensed for use in children. Some doses quoted are higher than those recommended by the manufacturers. Nebules® are not licensed for use in renal hyperkalaemia.

Salmeterol

■ **Aerosol inhaler:** 25 microgram per actuation.
■ **Breath-actuated inhaler:** 50 microgram per actuation.
■ **Dry powder inhaler:** 50 microgram per blister.

DOSAGE

Route	Age		Frequency (times daily)	Notes
	2–12 years	12–18 years		
Inhaled	< 4 years 25 microgram ≥ 4 years		2	<u>Preventor:</u> for regular use.

NOTES

■ Inhalers compatible with Volumatic® spacer device.

■ [L^E] Licensed for use ≥4 years of age.

Senna

[L^R]

■ **Tablets:** contain standardised senna ≡7.5mg total sennosides.
■ **Syrup:** one 5mL spoonful contains standardised senna extract ≡ 7.5mg total sennosides.

■ **Granules:** one 5mL level spoonful (2.73g) contains standardised senna ≡ 15mg total sennosides.

DOSAGE

Route	Age			Frequency	Notes
	1 month-2 years	2–12 years	12–18 years	(times daily)	
Oral (tablets)	-	<u><6 years</u> Not recommended <u>6-12 years</u> 1–2 tablets	2–4 tablets	1	
Oral (liquid)	0.5mL/kg	<u>2-6 years</u> 2.5–5mL <u>6-12 years</u> 5–10mL	10–20mL	1 1	

L[R]

DOSAGE continued

Route	Age			Frequency (times daily)	Notes
	1 month–2 years	2–12 years	12–18 years		
Oral (granules)	–	<6 years Not recommended 6–12 years 2.5–5mL	5–10mL	1	

NOTES

- **Administration: oral:** usually taken as a single dose at bedtime. May be taken in the morning by children. Granules may be stirred into a warm drink, sprinkled on food or eaten as they are.

- Onset of effect is usually within 24 hours.

- L[R] Syrup is licensed for use ≥2 years of age. Tablets and granules are licensed for use ≥6 years of age.

Sodium bicarbonate

L

- **Tablets:** 600mg (7.14mmol of sodium and bicarbonate).
- **Capsules:** 500mg (6mmol of sodium and bicarbonate).
- **Oral solution:** may be extemporaneously prepared.

- **Infusion:** 1.26% (0.15mmol of sodium and bicarbonate in 1mL), 500mL; 4.2% (0.5mmol of sodium and bicarbonate in 1mL), 10mL; 8.4% (1mmol of sodium and bicarbonate in 1mL), 10mL and 50mL disposable syringes and 200mL Polyfusor®.

DOSAGE

Indication	Route	Age				Frequency	Notes
		birth–1 month	1 month–2 years	2 – 12 years	12–18 years	(times daily)	
Metabolic acidosis	IV	← to correct acidosis → see intravenous fluid therapeutic guidelines section in *Medicines for Children*					
Renal acidosis	Oral	← 1–2mmol/kg/day →		← 70 mmol/m²/day →		1	Dose adjusted according to plasma bicarbonate level.
Renal hyperkalaemia	Slow IV	← 1mmol/kg (1mL/kg of 8.4%) →				single dose	
Resuscitation	Slow IV	← 1mL/kg of 8.4% initially followed by 0.5mL/kg of 8.4% if needed →					

NOTES

- **Administration: IV:** 1.26% may be given undiluted peripherally. Dilute other strengths with glucose 5%, glucose 10% or NaCl 0.9%. For peripheral administration, dilute the 8.4% to 1 in 10 and for central administration to 1 in 5. Caution is needed with renal patients – do not dilute with NaCl 0.9% due to the potential for hypernatraemia. Only used undiluted in an arrest or other emergency situations via a central line. Do not add to parenteral solutions containing calcium.

- Sodium component may increase fluid retention.

- Hypokalaemia may be exacerbated.

- 1.26% is an isotonic infusion.

- **Tablets (modified release):** 600mg (10mmol NaCl).
- **Capsules:** 300mg, 500mg, 600mg, 1g - all available as 'specials'.
- **Oral solutions:** 1mmol in 1mL, 2mmol in 1mL, 5mmol in 1mL – (30%) available as 'specials'.
- **Hypertonic solutions for nebulisation:** several strengths available as 'specials'.

- **Nasal drops:** 0.9% – manufactured 'special'.
- **Injection:** 30% (5mmol of sodium and chloride ions in 1mL), 10mL ampoules. 0.9% (0.15mmol of sodium and chloride ions in 1mL), several volumes of ampoule available.

DOSAGE

Sodium supplementation: dosage should be adjusted to individual needs, according to serum levels: as a guide;

Oral: <1 year – 500mg; 1–7 years – 1g; >7 years – 2–4g daily in divided doses.

IV: usual requirements as part of an intravenous feeding regimen are 2–5mmol/kg/day. Hyponatraemia; adjust the dose according to serum levels.

Chronic renal loss: orally: 1–2mmol Na$^+$/kg/day.

Nasal congestion in babies with rhinitis: instill 1–2 drops of NaCl 0.9% into each nostril before feeds.

To enhance mucoliary clearance in CF: 5-10% solutions nebulised twice daily before physiotherapy.

Supplementation for cystic fibrosis: CF patients may require sodium chloride supplements from April to September each year to replace losses in body fluids during warmer summer months. Patients should be supplemented if making trips abroad to warmer climates or if showing symptoms of salt depletion. Newly diagnosed infants may need regular sodium chloride supplements until the age of 1 year (then as above).

NOTES

- **Administration: IV:** NaCl 30% is hypertonic and should be diluted in a suitable infusion fluid of glucose, sodium chloride or PN before administration. **Nebulised:** hypertonic solutions nebulised via an

bronchoconstriction.

- The modified release tablets and the 0.9% injections and infusions are licensed for use in children and adults; all other preparations listed are

- **Tablets:** 250mg sodium fusidate (equivalent to 240mg fusidic acid).
- **Suspension:** 250mg fusidic acid in 5mL.
- **Intravenous infusion:** sodium fusidate 500mg (equivalent to 480mg fusidic acid) with 10mL vial of sterile phosphate-citrate buffer solution.

- **Cream:** fusidic acid BP 2% in a cream base.
- **Ointment:** sodium fusidate 2%.
- **Gel:** fusidic acid BP 2%.

DOSAGE

Route	Age				Frequency	Notes
	birth–1 month	1 month–2 years	2–12 years	12–18 years	(times daily)	
Oral	15mg/kg or 0.3mL/kg (fusidic acid)	<1 year as for neonate 1–2 years as for 2-5 years	2-5 years 250mg (5mL) (fusidic acid) 5-12 years 500mg (10mL) (fusidic acid)	750mg (15mL) (fusidic acid) or 500mg (2 tablets) (sodium fusidate)	3 3	Treatment of asymptomatic *S. aureus* isolates or minor exacerbations in cystic fibrosis patients. For cutaneous infections 12–18 years 1 tablet twice daily is the standard treatment.
IV infusion	←	6-7mg/kg (sodium fusidate)	→	DOSE BY WEIGHT <u><50kg</u> 6-7mg/kg (sodium fusidate) DOSE BY AGE <u>>50kg</u> 500mg (sodium fusidate)	3 3	Doses may be doubled in severe infections.

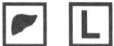

DOSAGE continued

Route	Age				Frequency (times daily)	Notes
	birth–1 month	1 month–2 years	2–12 years	12–18 years		
Topical	← Apply to the affected area →				3–4	Uncovered lesions; less frequent application may be adequate for covered lesions

NOTES

■ **Administration: IV infusion:** to reconstitute, dissolve the contents of 1 vial containing 500mg sodium fusidate powder (equivalent to 480mg of fusidic acid) in the 10mL buffer provided. Further dilute to 1mg in 1mL with NaCl 0.9% or another suitable infusion fluid (glucose 5%, compound sodium lactate, sodium lactate, sodium chloride 0.18%/glucose 4%, KCL 0.3%/ glucose 5%). The diluted fluid should be infused over at least 6 hours if a superficial vein is employed or over 2 hours via a central venous line. If additional antibacterial therapy is to be employed, it is recommended that for parenteral administration, separate infusion fluids be used. Sodium fusidate is physically incompatible with infusion fluids containing 20% or more of glucose, lipid infusions and peritoneal dialysis fluids. Precipitation may occur in dilutions which result in a pH of less than 7.4.

■ ▶ Periodic liver function tests should be carried out when high oral doses are used, when the drug is given for prolonged periods and in patients with liver dysfunction.

■ **Oral liquid:** 5mg in 5mL.

DOSAGE

Route	Age			Frequency (times daily)	Notes
	1 month–2 years	2–12 years	12–18 years		
Oral	–	2–5 years 2.5mL	5–15mL	1	Take at night
		5–10 years 2.5–5mL		1	
		≥10 years 5–15mL		1	

NOTES
■ **Administration: oral:** may be diluted with purified water.

■ Onset of action is 10-14 hours.

Sodium valproate

■ **Tablets (crushable):** 100mg.
■ **Tablets (enteric coated):** 200mg, 500mg.
■ **Tablets (modified release):** 200mg, 300mg, 500mg.

■ **Oral liquid & oral syrup:** 200mg in 5mL.
■ **Suppositories:** 300mg.
■ **Injection:** 400mg vial (with 4mL ampoule of Water for Injections).

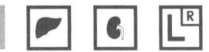

DOSAGE

Route	Age				Frequency (times daily)	Notes
	*birth– 1 month	1 month– 2 years	2–12 years	12–18 years		
Oral	20mg/kg	–		–	1	Starting dose
	–	← 5-7.5mg/kg →		300mg	2	
	10–20mg/kg	← 12.5-15mg/kg →		500mg-1g	2	<u>Usual target maintenance dose</u> (doses up to 20mg/kg twice daily have been used and up to 30mg/kg twice daily has been used in the treatment of infantile spasms).
Oral m/r tablets	–	← 10-15mg/kg →		600mg	1	Starting dose
	–	← 25-30mg/kg →		1-2g	1	Usual target maintenance dose.
IV bolus over 3–5 minutes	← 10mg/kg →				2	Introduction, if oral not possible. For established therapy substitute IV for oral at same dose.
IV infusion	–	←20-40mg/kg/day →		maximum 2.5g/day	continuous	Following a bolus of 10mg/kg.
Rectal	← as for oral →					

*Experience in the neonatal use of sodium valproate is extremely limited.

NOTES

■ **Administration: oral:** crushable tablets are scored and may be halved and/or crushed. **IV:** adding 4 mL Water for Injections to 400 mg powder produces 95 mg/mL; administer by direct injection or diluted in glucose 5%, NaCl 0.9% or glucose/ saline. Dilutions stable for 24 hours.

■ Contra-indicated in active liver disease and family history of liver dysfunction, especially if drug related. Counsel on recognition of liver adverse effects. Measure pre-treatment liver function in children under 3 years of age with severe cryptogenic epilepsy (featuring myoclonic seizures), additional learning difficulties and if receiving another antiepileptic. Monitor liver function of all patients during therapy if clinically indicated.

■ Counsel on recognition of haematological adverse effects. Monitor blood tests of all patients during therapy if clinically indicated. If doses greater than 40mg/kg/day are required monitor biochemistry and blood counts. Full blood count advised before surgery. For more information refer to the manufacturer's SPC.

■ Dose should be reduced in severe renal failure.

■ Interactions with many other anticonvulsants; consult *Medicines for Children* or product literature for more details.

■ The suppositories are not licensed for use in the UK. They may be obtained on a named patient basis via IDIS World Medicines.

Spironolactone

■ **Tablets:** 25mg, 50mg, 100mg.

■ **Suspensions:** 5mg in 5mL, 10mg in 5mL, 25mg in 5mL, 50mg in 5mL and 100mg in 5mL.

DOSAGE

Route	Age				Frequency	Notes
	birth–1 month	1 month–2 years	2–12 years	12–18 years	(times daily)	
Oral	← 500 microgram/kg–1.5mg/kg →			25–50mg	2	Dose should be adjusted on the basis of response and tolerance. The total daily dose may, if necessary, be given as one dose or divided into more than 2 doses. Plasma potassium levels should be monitored. In children, doses up to 9mg/kg/day have been used with careful monitoring in resistant ascites.

SPIRONOLACTONE SHOULD NOT ROUTINELY BE ADMINISTERED CONCURRENTLY WITH POTASSIUM SPARING DIURETICS OR POTASSIUM SUPPLEMENTS AS HYPERKALAEMIA MAY BE INDUCED.

NOTES

■ Contra-indicated in patients with creatinine clearance <30ml/min/1.73m². Fluid and electrolyte status should be regularly monitored in patients with significant renal impairment. Plasma potassium levels should be monitored.

■ Fluid and electrolyte status should be regularly monitored in patients with significant hepatic impairment. Although the dose of spironolactone does not generally need to be reduced in hepatic dysfunction such patients should be carefully monitored as hepatic coma may be precipitated in susceptible patients.

■ The oral suspensions are available as 'specials' from Rosemont and as such are unlicensed.

■ To convert to IV potassium canrenoate dose, multiply spironolactone dose by 1.45.

- **Tablets:** 1g.
- **Oral suspension:** 1g in 5mL.

DOSAGE

Route	Age				Frequency (times daily)	Notes
	birth–1 month	1 month–2 years	2–12 years	12–18 years		
Oral	–	250mg	500mg	1g	4–6	

NOTES

- **Administration: oral:** tablets may be crushed or dispersed in water. Caution with administration via nasogastric or gastrostomy tubes which can become blocked. Doses should be taken before meals, and spread throughout the waking hours.

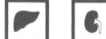

- **Tablets:** 500mg.
- **Tablets (enteric coated):** 500mg.
- **Suspension:** 250mg in 5mL.
- **Suppositories:** 500mg.
- **Enema:** 3g in 100mL.

DOSAGE

Indication	Route	Age		Frequency (times daily)	Notes
		2–12 years	12–18 years		
JIA	Oral	← 5mg/kg →		2	1st week
		← 10mg/kg →		2	2nd week
		← 20mg/kg →		2	3rd week
		← 20–25mg/kg →		2	maintenance dose
		Maximum 2g/day	Maximum 3g/day		
Ulcerative colitis/ Crohn's disease	Oral	10–15mg/kg		4–6	Acute attack. Reduce dose by 50% for maintenance treatment. Maximum dose 60mg/kg/day.
			1–2g	4	
	Rectal suppository	2-4 years ⅓ adult dose 5-7 years ½ adult dose 8-12 years	2 suppositories	2	In the morning and at bedtime, preferably after defecation. 5-7 years use 1 suppository twice daily. 8-12 years use 1 suppository in the morning and 2 in the evening, or vice versa.

DOSAGE continued

Indication	Route	Age		Frequency (times daily)	Notes
		2–12 years	12–18 years		
Ulcerative colitis/ Crohn's disease	Rectal enema	2-7 years ¹/₃-¹/₂ adult dose 7-12 years ¹/₂-³/₄ adult dose	One enema	1	Preferably at bedtime. A proportion of the enema may be used to administer smaller doses.

NOTES

- 🖊 🄒 Patients with renal or hepatic disease should be treated with caution. Liver function tests should be performed at the start of treatment and monthly thereafter.

- Full blood counts should be performed initially, and monthly thereafter. An immediate blood count should be carried out if neutropenia or thrombocytopenia are suspected due to symptoms such as sore throat, glossitis, buccal ulceration, easy bruising or bleeding. If any abnormal results are found, treatment should be withheld and discussed with the clinician responsible for the child's care. In patients with G6PD deficiency, monitor for signs of haemolytic anaemia.

- Severe nausea or dizziness may necessitate dosage reduction or drug withdrawal.

- 🄛 Plain (uncoated) tablets, suspension and suppositories are licensed for use ≥2 years of age for ulcerative colitis and Crohn's disease but not for arthritis. The enteric coated tablets are licensed for ulcerative colitis and Crohn's disease in adults and children ≥2 years of age but for arthritis in adults only. The enema is not licensed for use in children.

■ **Tablets:** 50mg, 100mg.

■ **Injection:** (as succinate) 12mg in 1mL, 0.5mL pre-filled syringe and auto-injector.

■ **Nasal spray:** 20mg in 0.1mL unit-dose spray device.

DOSAGE

Route	Age		Frequency	Notes
	2-12 years	12-18 years		
Oral	6-10 years 25mg 10-12 years 50mg	50-100mg	single dose	Dose may be repeated if migraine recurs. Maximum of 300mg in 24 hours. If patient does not respond, they should not take a second dose for the same attack.
SC	10-12 years 6mg	6mg	single dose	Dose may be repeated once, after not less than 1 hour, if migraine recurs. Maximum of 12mg in 24 hours. If patient does not respond, they should not take a second dose for the same attack.
Intranasally	–	20mg	single dose	Dose may be repeated once, after not less than 2 hours, if migraine recurs. Maximum of 40mg in 24 hours. If patient does not respond, they should not take a second dose for the same attack.

NOTES

■ **Administration: Oral:** 50mg tablet can be halved, however it has a very bitter taste. The remaining unused half should be discarded.
Intranasal: 1 spray into 1 nostril; can give a bitter taste by this route.

■ **CSM advice:** discontinue if intense pain in chest – may be due to coronary vasoconstriction or anaphylaxis.

Surfactants (natural)

■ **Injection:** 120mg in 1.5mL, 240mg in 3mL as poractant alfa.

■ **Injection:** 200mg in 8mL as beractant.

DOSAGE

Product	Route	Dosage			Frequency (times daily)	Notes
		birth–1 month				
Poractant alfa	Intra-tracheal	←	200mg/kg (2.5mL/kg)	→	single bolus	<u>Initial dose.</u> Followed by two further doses of 100mg/kg after 12 and 24 hours if necessary.
Beractant	Intra-tracheal	←	100mg/kg (4mL/kg)	→	single bolus	Up to 3 further doses of 100mg/kg can be given, at intervals of not less than 6 hours, within the next 48 hours.

NOTES

■ **Administration: intra-tracheal:** pre-oxygenate baby before administration; ventilate during administration.

■ Ⓛ Licensed for use in preterm infants greater than 700g birthweight.

Surfactant (synthetic)

■ **Injection:** 108mg powder vial with 8mL preservative-free sterile water – as colfosceril palmitate.

DOSAGE

Route	Dosage		Frequency	Notes
	birth–1 month		(times daily)	
Intra-tracheal	← 67.5mg/kg →		single dose	Give over 4 minutes. A further dose of 67.5mg/kg can be given after 12 hours if the baby is still ventilated.

NOTES

■ **Administration: intra-tracheal:** pre-oxygenate baby before administration;

■ Ⓛ Licensed for use in newborn infants.

■ **Injection:** 200mg, 400mg vials (with diluent).

DOSAGE

Newborn infant

Route	Age		Frequency (times daily)	Notes
	birth–1 month			
IV	16mg/kg		single dose	Loading dose, then 24 hours later start the Maintenance dose.
	8mg/kg		1	

Child

Route	Age			Frequency (times daily)	Notes
	1 month-2 years	2–12 years	12–18 years		
IV	←	10mg/kg	→	2	Give this dose for 3 doses then as outlined below for moderate or severe infections. Maximum single dose 400mg ie ≥40kg body weight dose is 400mg.
IM/IV	←	10mg/kg	→	1	Severe infections, neutropenic patients and cystic fibrosis patients. Maximum single dose 400mg ie ≥40kg body weight dose is 400mg.
	←	6mg/kg	→	1	Moderate infections. Maximum single dose 200mg ie ≥34kg body weight dose is 200mg.
Oral	←	10mg/kg	→	2	Unlicensed route in treatment of pseudomembranous colitis.

Child continued

Route	Age			Frequency	Notes
	1 month–2 years	2–12 years	12–18 years		
Intra-ventricular	5mg	10mg	20mg	once daily initially	Frequency of administration may reduce to alternate days if there is a good response. Unlicensed route; very limited experience. Administer in appropriate volume of NaCl 0.9%.
Intra-peritoneal	Concentration of 20mg/L per bag for first week then alternate bags for second week then overnight only during third week.				Treatment of peritonitis in CAPD Use single IV loading dose first.

 Dose adjustment in renal impairment – Dose reduction is not required until the 4th day of treatment. Monitor urea and creatinine.

Degree of renal impairment	Dose
Mild	Half of the daily dose
Moderate to severe	One third of the daily dose

NOTES

■ **Administration: IV/IM:** the injection vial should be reconstituted with the

400mg or 200mg in 3mL as excess is included in the vial. Roll the vial gently until the powder is completely dissolved. Excessive agitation may lead to

IV injection or by IV infusion over 30 minutes. Compatible with NaCl 0.9%, glucose 5% and glucose 4%/NaCl 0.18%; should not be mixed with aminoglycosides.

■ Licensed for use in all ages, however, in newborn infants teicoplanin is only licensed for administration by infusion over 30 minutes.

Temazepam (controlled drug)

■ **Tablets:** 10mg, 20mg.
■ **Gel filled capsules:** 10mg, 15mg, 20mg, 30mg.
■ **Oral solution:** 10mg in 5mL.

DOSAGE

Route	Age				Frequency	Notes
	birth–1 month	1 month–2 years	2–12 years	12–18 years		
Oral	–	←——— 1mg/kg ———→		20–30mg	single dose	Administer one hour prior to procedure or surgery.

NOTES

■ Avoid in CNS depression, coma, acute pulmonary insufficiency, myasthenia gravis and sleep apnoea syndrome.

■ In severe renal impairment use reduced doses (increased cerebral sensitivity). Dose reduction is not necessary in mild to moderate renal impairment.

■ Dose reduction is not necessary in liver disease. Caution in severe liver disease; may precipitate coma.

L[R]

- **Tablets:** 5mg.
- **Tablets (modified release):** 7.5mg.
- **Syrup:** 1.5mg in 5mL.
- **Aerosol inhaler:** 250 microgram per actuation.

- **Dry powder inhaler:** 500 microgram per actuation.
- **Nebuliser solution:** 5mg in 2mL, 10mg in 1mL, 20mL.
- **Injection:** 500 microgram in 1mL; 1mL & 5mL ampoules.

DOSAGE

Route	Age			Frequency	Notes
	1 month–2 years	2–12 years	12–18 years	(times daily)	
Oral	75 microgram/kg	**DOSE BY WEIGHT** ≤7 years 75 microgram/kg **DOSE BY AGE** ≥7 years 2.5mg	2.5–5mg	3 2–3	
Oral m/r tablets	–	–	7.5mg	2	
Aerosol inhaler	← 250 – 500 microgram →			4–6	Reliever: doses are given as required. Higher doses have been used in acute asthma

Route	Age			Frequency	Notes
	1 month-2 years	2-12 years	12-18 years	(times daily)	
Dry powder inhaler	–	>5 years ◀—1 inhalation (500 microgram)—▶		4	Reliever.
Nebuliser	2.5-5mg	≤5 years 2.5-5mg ▔▔▔ >5 years 5-10mg	10mg	single dose	Reliever. Doses are given as required; up to 8 times daily if necessary or 12 times daily under hospital supervision.
Injection SC/IM/ Slow IV bolus	–	10 microgram/kg (maximum 300 microgram/dose)	250-500 microgram	single dose	Emergency use if nebuliser not available. Repeat up to 4 times daily.
IV infusion (loading dose)	◀— 2-4 microgram/kg —▶			single dose	The optimum therapeutic dose in children is still empiric. The doses vary considerably depending on the reference source. Doses up to 5 times those given here have been used.
IV infusion (maintenance)	◀— 1-10 microgram/kg/hour —▶			continuous	

NOTES

■ **Administration: oral:** 5mg tablets are scored and can be halved; m/r tablets should be swallowed whole. **Nebulisation:** nebuliser solution can be diluted with NaCl 0.9% or mixed with ipratropium bromide or budesonide nebuliser solutions. **Inhaled aerosol:** inhalers can be used with a Nebuhaler® spacer device and mask for infants and young children.

■ Licensed for use in all ages, however some preparations are only suitable for older children. Some doses and dosage intervals stated are higher than recommended by the manufacturer. The injection is only licensed for use in newborn infants if given by infusion.

Tetracaine (amethocaine) – Ametop®

■ **Gel:** tetracaine 4%, 1.5g tube – Ametop®

DOSAGE

Route	Age				Frequency	Notes
	birth–1 month	1 month–2 years	2–12 years	12–18 years		
Topical	Not recommended	← the contents of one tube (approximately 1g) →			single application	This quantity is sufficient to anaesthetise an area up to 30cm² (6 x 5cm). Smaller areas of anaesthetised skin may be adequate in infants and small children.

NOTES

■ **Administration:** The required amount of gel is applied to the centre of the area to be anaesthetised and covered with an occlusive dressing. Anaesthesia will be adequate for venepuncture after 30 minutes and for venous cannulation after 45 minutes. Anaesthesia remains for 4-6 hours in most patients after a single application.

■ Use with caution in children <1 month of age as metabolic pathways may not be fully developed.

■ Tetracaine should not be applied to inflamed, traumatised or highly vascular areas, the eyes or ears.

■ It is rapidly absorbed from mucous membranes and should never be used to provide anaesthesia for bronchoscopy or cystography.

■ 🄻ᴱ Licensed for use ≥1 month of age. Not recommended for premature infants and infants <1 month of age.

Theophylline

🄻ᴿ

■ **Tablets (normal release):** 125mg.
■ **Tablets (modified release):** 175mg, 200mg, 250mg, 300mg, 400mg.

■ **Capsules (modified release):** 60mg, 125mg, 250mg.
■ **Oral liquid:** 60mg in 5mL.

DOSAGE
Child

Indication	Route/ Preparation	Age			Frequency (times daily)	Notes
		1 month–2 years	2–12 years	12–18 years		
Asthma	Oral/ normal release preparations	>6 months 5mg/kg	← 5mg/kg →		3–4	Starting dose. Adjust dose according to clinical response and plasma levels.
	Oral/ modified release preparations	>6 months 12mg/kg	2–7 years 12mg/kg	8mg/kg	2	Maximum 500mg per dose. Starting dose. Adjust dose according to clinical response and plasma levels.
			8–12 years 10mg/kg		2	

NOTES

■ **Administration: oral:** modified release tablets should be swallowed whole or halved using the score line and each half swallowed whole. They must not be crushed or chewed. Normal release tablets are soluble in water. Capsules can be opened and the contents sprinkled onto soft food – must be swallowed without chewing. Do not interchange brands.

■ Consult *Medicines for Children* for details of therapeutic drug monitoring.

■ L^R Asthma therapy – use <2 years of age is an unlicensed indication. See *Medicines for Children* for individual product details.

■ **Injection:** 10,000 units in 1mL; 2500 units in 0.25mL, 3500 units in 0.35mL, 4500 units in 0.45mL prefilled syringes and 2mL vial .

■ **Injection:** 20,000 units in 1mL; 10,000 units in 0.5mL, 14,000 units in 0.7mL, 18,000 units in 0.9mL prefilled syringes and 2mL vial.

DOSAGE

Indication	Route	Age			Frequency	Notes
		1 month–2 years	2–12 years	12–18 years	(times daily)	
Prophylaxis of venous thrombo-embolism	SC	←	50 units /kg	→	1	
Treatment of deep vein thrombosis and pulmonary embolism	SC	←	175 units/kg	→	1	Used for at least 6 days. Tinzaparin therapy docs not require routine monitoring in patients with normal renal and hepatic function.

Experience of the use in children is very limited.

NOTES

Care should be taken when tinazaparin is administered to patients with severe liver insufficiency who are undergoing general or orthopaedic surgery. Care should also be taken when tinazaparin is administered to patients with severe liver insufficiency during haemodialysis.

Patients with severe renal impairment may require reduced doses. Both trough and peak anti-Xa activity must be monitored on a daily basis.

Take a trough immediately prior to the next dose and a peak level 3-4 hours after the dose. Trough values should be around 0.2 units/mL and peak values should be between 0.8-1 unit/mL. Care should be taken when tinazaparin is administered to patients with severe renal insufficiency who are undergoing general or orthopaedic surgery.

As different low molecular weight heparins may not be equivalent, alternative products should not be substituted during a course of treatment.

Tobramycin

■ **Injection:** 20mg in 2mL, 40mg in 1mL, 80mg in 2mL.
■ **Oral solution:** various strengths can be extemporaneously prepared.

■ **Nebuliser solution:** 300mg in 5mL (preservative-free).

Many dose regimens exist; those outlined below are generally accepted initial doses and dose adjustments should be made in the light of serum concentration measurement.

DOSAGE

Extended dosing regimen

Newborn infant (birth to 1 month)

Route	Postconceptional age	Dose	Dose frequency	Notes
IV	<32 weeks	4–5mg/kg	36 hourly	Plasma samples usually taken around the third dose aiming for 1 hour post dose (peak) of 5–10mg/L and a pre dose (trough) level of <2mg/L If there is no change in the dosage regimen or renal function repeat levels every 3-4 days.
	>32 weeks	4–5mg/kg	24 hourly	

Postconceptional age = gestational age plus postnatal age.
Neonates presenting with patent ductus arteriosus (PDA), prolonged hypoxia or treated with indometacin (indomethacin) may have impaired elimination of tobramycin due to reduced glomerular filtration rate (GFR) and increase in dosage interval may be necessary.

Divided daily dose regimen

Child

Route	Age			Frequency (times daily)	Notes
	1 month–2 years	2–12 years	12–18 years		
IV/IM	← 2.5mg/kg →		1–2mg/kg	3	Severe infection. Plasma samples usually taken around the third or fourth dose aiming for a pre dose (trough) level of <2mg/L and a 1 hour post dose (peak) level of 5–10mg/L.
IV	← 4mg/kg →			3	Starting dose in cystic fibrosis. Monitor levels after third dose. Aim for a pre dose (trough) <2mg/L and 1 hour post dose (peak) level of 8–12mg/L

In renal impairment monitor levels and increase the dosing interval keeping the dose the same as normal or adjust dose and dosing interval. Two sample regimens are outlined below.

Regimen 1

Degree of renal impairment	Dose adjustment
Mild	75% of a dose 12 hourly
Moderate	50% of a dose 12 hourly
Severe	50% of a dose 24 hourly

Regimen 2

Creatinine clearance (mL/minute/1.73m²)	Dosage interval (hours) (dose stays the same)
40–70	12
20–40	18
10–20	24
5–10	36
<5	48

Child continued

Route	Age			Frequency (times daily)	Notes
	1 month-2 years	2-12 years	12-18 years		
Nebulised for cystic fibrosis patients	–	≥6 years 300mg	300mg	2	TOBI preservative-free solution. Alternating 28 days on and 28 days off. Licensed product is nebulised treatment of choice.
	40mg	≤8 years 80mg	160mg	2	Injection - not licensed for nebulisation. Seek advice from pharmacy department before prescribing. Intravenous preparations must be preservative-free (phenol-free) solutions. Dilute to 4mL with NaCl 0.9%.
		≥8 years 160mg		2	
Oral	20mg	≤5 years 20mg	80mg	4	Selective decontamination of digestive tract (with colistin and amphotericin). Unlicensed and limited experience of use.
		5-12 years 40mg		4	

Single daily dose regimen
Child

Route	Age			Frequency (times daily)	Notes (monitoring)
	1 month–2 years	**2–12 years**	**12–18 years**		
IV	←	7mg/kg	→	1	Plasma samples are usually taken at 18-24 hours after the first dose aiming for a level <1mg/L If the levels are >1mg/L then the dosing interval is normally increased by 12 hours. 1 hour post dose (peak) levels can be taken with a target range of 16-20mg/L If there is no change in the dosage regimen or in renal function repeat levels every 3-4 days.

Pre-dose levels must be monitored in children with impaired renal function.

NOTES

■ **Administration:** slow IV injection over 3–5 minutes injected neat or diluted in NaCl 0.9% or glucose 5%. IV infusion over 30–60 minutes for high dose 'child – single daily dose regimen' in an appropriate volume of NaCl 0.9% or glucose 5%. Avoid mixing with penicillins, cephalosporins or erythromycin. **Nebulised: Nebulised using the nebuliser solution:** administer the contents of one unit over a 15 minute period, using a hand-held PARI LC PLUS reusable nebuliser. Administer after physiotherapy and bronchodilators. Tobramycin must not be mixed in the nebuliser with any other drugs. **Nebulised using the injection solution:** optimum nebulisation volume 4mL – make up to volume with NaCl 0.9%. Administer after physiotherapy and bronchodilators. An active venturi nebuliser system with outlet is recommended so exhaled antibiotic can be discharged via a window otherwise an effective filter system should be used. Tobramycin must not be mixed in the nebuliser with any other drugs.

solution; parenteral routes licensed in all ages. Nebuliser solution is licensed for use > 6 years of age.

■ Not licensed for oral administration or nebulisation using the injection

Topiramate

■ **Tablets:** 25mg, 50mg, 100mg, 200mg.

■ **Capsules:** 15mg, 25mg, 50mg.

DOSAGE

Route	Age				Frequency (times daily)	Notes
	birth–1 month	1 month–2 years	2–12 years	12–18 years		
Oral	–	← 500 microgram/kg →		25mg	1	Usual starting dose.
	–	← 2–4.5mg/kg →		100–200mg	2	Usual target maintenance dose. Doses up to 6mg/kg twice daily have been used.

NOTES

■ **Administration: Oral:** can be taken with or without food. Crushed tablets are very bitter but can be mixed with strong tasting food or liquid. Capsules may be opened and the beads mixed with soft food; beads should not be chewed.

■ **Dose adjustment:** Use starting dose for 2 weeks then increase dose every 2 weeks taking at least 6 weeks to reach maintenance dose.

■ Use with caution in renal failure titrating dose and intervals between dose adjustments to efficacy and side-effects. Supplemental doses required after dialysis.

■ May increase plasma *phenytoin* levels. *Carbamazepine* and *phenytoin* may decrease topiramate levels.

■ Licensed for adjunctive therapy >2 years of age. Licensed >6years of age as monotherapy for newly diagnosed epilepsy.

■ **Tablets:** 100mg, 200mg. ■ **Suspension:** 50mg in 5mL.

DOSAGE
Newborn infant

Route	Age	Frequency	Notes
	birth to 1 month	(times daily)	
Oral	3mg/kg then 2mg/kg	loading dose then 2	Treatment dose.
Oral	2mg/kg	once (in the evening)	Prophylaxis dose.

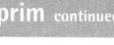

DOSAGE continued

Child

Route	Age			Frequency (times daily)	Notes
	1 month–2 years	2–12 years	12–18 years		
Oral	←	4mg/kg	→	2	Treatment dose. Maximum single dose 200mg i.e. ≥ 50kg body weight dose is 200mg.
Oral	←	2mg/kg	→	once (at night)	Prophylaxis dose.

🝗 : Dose adjustment in renal impairment – reduce dose frequency.

<u>Moderate impairment:</u> normal dose for 3 days then 50% of dose 12 hourly.

<u>Severe impairment:</u> 50% of dose 12 hourly.

Should not be given to dialysis patients unless plasma concentration can be measured.

NOTES
- Avoid in the 1st trimester of pregnancy as animal studies have shown teratogenic potential and it is a folate antagonist.

- 🆛 Licensed in children >6 weeks of age. In neonates, license states 'use under careful medical supervision'.

■ **Tablet:** 150mg, 300mg.
■ **Capsule:** 250mg.

■ **Suspension:** 250mg in 5mL.
■ **Powder:** can be extemporaneously prepared.

DOSAGE

Route	Age				Frequency (times daily)	Notes
	birth–1 month	1 month–2 years	2–12 years	12–18 years		
Oral	← 5-10mg/kg →				2-3	Maximum total daily dose of 45mg/kg/**day**.
Oral for cystic fibrosis patients	–	← 10mg/kg →			2	To improve bile flow in cystic fibrosis patients with liver impairment. **Total daily dose** may be given in three divided doses.

NOTES

■ **Administration: oral:** the last dose of the day should be taken in the late evening to counteract the rise in biliary cholesterol saturation which occurs in the early hours of the morning. Take with food; this is especially useful with the late evening dose as it helps to maintain bile flow overnight. Starting at a lower dose initially, increasing to the final dose over about 2 weeks, can help to prevent problems with abdominal discomfort, which may occur.

■ Should not be used during pregnancy.

■ Only one brand of 250mg capsules is licensed for use in children (Ursofalk®) and only for treatment of primary biliary cirrhosis and the dissolution of radiolucent gallstones in patients with a functioning gallbladder; other preparations and indications are unlicensed in children.

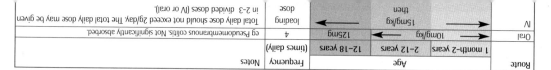

■ **Capsule:** 125mg, 250mg. ■ **Injection:** 500mg, 1g vials.

DOSAGE

Newborn infant

Route	*Postconceptional age	Dose	Frequency (times daily)
IV	<28 weeks	15mg/kg	1
	29-35 weeks	15mg/kg	2
	>35 weeks	15mg/kg	3
Intrathecal	All newborn infants	2.5 – 5mg	1

*postconceptional age = gestational plus postnatal age

Child

Route	Age — 1 month-2 years	2-12 years	12-18 years	Frequency (times daily)	Notes
Oral	← 10mg/kg →		125mg	4	eg Pseudomembranous colitis. Not significantly absorbed.
IV	← 15mg/kg then →		loading dose	Total daily dose should not exceed 2g/day. The total daily dose may be given in 2-3 divided doses (IV or oral).

DOSAGE continued

Route	Age			Frequency	Notes
	1 month-2 years	2-12 years	12-18 years	(times daily)	
IV for cystic fibrosis patients	←	10mg/kg	→	4	Starting dose. Amend according to levels. Monitor levels after third dose. Trough level of 5-10mg/L is acceptable and up to 15mg/L may be preferred in severe infections. Post dose (peak) level 1 hour after completion of infusion of 18-25mg/L Always check local policy.
Intrathecal	5mg	≤4 years 5mg 4-12 years 10mg	≤15 years 10mg >15 years 20mg	single single	Patients with enlarged ventricles require higher doses. Adjust dose according to CSF levels after 3-4 days. Aim for trough level of<10mg/L.

 Dose adjustment in renal impairment, Avoid parenteral route if possible in renal impairment. Dose is reduced according to blood levels. In anuric patients, a loading dose of 15mg/kg then a dose every several days may be sufficient. In peritoneal dialysis add vancomycin to dialysis fluids either as 20mg/L in each bag for 5 days or 100mg/L in one bag only per day for 5 days.

NOTES

■ **Administration: IV:** intermittent infusion is the preferred method of administration though continuous infusion has been used when intermittent infusion is not feasible. On reconstitution, 500mg powder displaces 0.3mL. For intravenous administration add 9.7mL Water for Injections to give a 50mg in 1mL solution. This should be further diluted with NaCl 0.9% or glucose 5% to give 5mg in 1mL which is infused over at least 1 hour. In fluid restricted patients maximum concentration is 10mg in 1mL, infused centrally over at least 1 hour.
Oral: the injection may be given orally. Common flavouring syrups may be added to the solution at the time of administration. Solutions of the parenteral powder intended for oral use may be stored in a fridge (2-8°C) for 96 hours.

■ Pharmacokinetics: requires blood level monitoring. Approximate time to steady state is 1-2 days. Suggested sampling times for levels at 4th dose: trough – immediately prior to next dose; peak – 1 hour after completion of infusion. Therapeutic levels – trough 5-10mg/L.; peak 18-26mg/L. CSF level monitoring – take trough sample immediately prior to next dose. Level should be <10mg/L.

■ Licensed for use in all ages except for administration via the intrathecal route which is unlicensed.

■ **Tablets:** 500mg.

■ **Sachets:** 500mg (powder to be dissolved).

DOSAGE

Route	Age				Frequency (times daily)	Notes
	birth–1 month	1 month–2 years	2–12 years	12–18 years		
Oral	← 15-20mg/kg →			1g	2	Usual starting dose
	← 30-40mg/kg →			1-1.5g	2	Usual target maintenance dose
	← 15-25mg/kg →		-	-	2	Infantile spasms Usual starting dose
	← 40-50mg/kg →		-	-	2	Infantile spasms Usual target maintenance dose. Maximum dose of 75mg/kg twice daily.

NOTES

■ **Administration: oral:** may be taken before or after food. Dissolve contents of sachet in water or soft drink, a proportion can be measured to obtain smaller doses. Tablets can be crushed and dispersed in liquid or soft food.

■ **C** Reduce dose if creatinine clearance is <60 mL/min/1.73m^2.

■ May exacerbate myoclonic seizures.

■ Monitor for peripheral constriction of visual fields.

■ **Dose adjustment:** increase to maintenance dose over 2-3 weeks except for infantile spasms when the maintenance dose should be reached in 5-7 days. Warn not to cease therapy without advice, withdraw gradually.

■ **Tablets:** 50mg, 200mg.
■ **Suspension:** 500mg in 5mL.

■ **Injection:** 100mg in 1mL; 2mL ampoule.

DOSAGE
Newborn infant

Route	Age		Frequency	Notes
	birth–1 month			
Oral	10mg/kg		once daily	Nutritional deficiency.
Oral	100mg/kg		once daily	Abetalipoproteinaemia.
IM	20mg/kg		single dose	Neonatal prophylaxis, given at birth to babies weighing less than 1kg or 1.5kg in some UK neonatal units.

DOSAGE
Child

Route	Age			Frequency	Notes
	1 month-2 years	2-12 years	12-18 years		
Oral	<1 year 50mg ≥1 year 100mg	100mg	200mg	once daily once daily	Supplement in cystic fibrosis.
Oral	←	50–100mg/kg	→	once daily	Abetalipoproteinaemia
Oral	150–200mg/kg	-	-	once daily	Initial dose to prevent deficiency secondary to chronic cholestasis. Increase to keep vitamin E/lipid ratio >0.6. May need up to 200mg/kg/day.
IM	10mg/kg (maximum 100mg)	-	-	once a month	

NOTES

■ [L̃] injection available on a named patient basis from John Bell and Croydon. Tablets and suspension are licensed for use in all ages.

■ Premature infants weighing less than 1.5kg treated with oral vitamin E have a higher rate of necrotizing enterocolitis.

Phytomenadione (vitamin K1)
- **Tablets:** 10mg – Konakion®.
- **Capsules:** 500microgram, 1mg – Orakay®.
- **Injection:** 1mg in 0.5mL – Konakion®Neonatal.
- **Injection (mixed micelles formulation):** 2mg in 0.2mL – Konakion®MM

Paediatric; 10mg in 1mL – Konakion®MM.

Menadiol sodium diphosphate (vitamin K analogue).
- **Tablets:** 10mg.

DOSAGE

Neonates and babies: vitamin K deficiency bleeding Prophylaxis: current practice continues to vary widely throughout the UK; please refer to local policy. See also *Medicines for Children* for further details. **Treatment:** 1mg IV repeated at 8 hourly intervals if necessary.

Child

Indication	Route	Age			Frequency (times daily)	Notes
		1 month–2 years	2–12 years	12–18 years		
Antidote to anticoagulants	IV	← 15–30 microgram/kg* →			single dose	Seek expert advice before prescribing Measure INR (venous) after 2-6 hours and again the next day.
Other indications	Oral/ IM	← 300 microgram/kg →		10mg	1	Use water soluble preparation for oral supplementation in fat malabsorption.

NOTES

■ **Administration: oral:** menadiol tablets may be crushed with food or dissolved in water (NB the excipients are not soluble). Konakion® tablets are to be chewed or allowed to dissolve slowly in the mouth. Konakion® MM Paediatric can be given orally. After breaking the ampoule open, 0.2mL (2mg) of solution should be withdrawn into the syringe and the plunger then depressed to dispense the contents directly into the baby's mouth. Orakay® capsules – only the capsule contents are given by cutting the side tube of the capsule and expressing the contents directly into the baby's mouth or into a feed.

IV or IM: Konakion® Neonatal is for IM injection; not recommended to be given by the IV route and should not be diluted. Konakion® MM Paediatric can be injected neat or into the lower part of an infusion set (of glucose 5%). It should not be mixed with other parenteral medications or diluted (but in practice the small volume may necessitate dilution in order to administer the dose; in which case glucose 5% should be used). Konakion® MM is for IV injection (neat solution) or for IV infusion; when it should be diluted with 55mL of glucose 5%.

■ 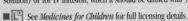 See *Medicines for Children* for full licensing details.

■ *A full dose of Vitamin K (300 micrograms/kg) will completely reverse the anticoagulant effect and make warfarin very difficult to reintroduce for up to 2 weeks (warfarin resistance).

Nutrition Tables
Special Infant Formulae

SPECIAL INFANT FORMULA

Composition per 100ml

Name of formula	Energy/100mL		Protein	g/100mL	Carbohydrate	g/100mL	Fat	g/100mL
	kcal	KJ						
Protein hydrolysate: Nutramigen is ACBS prescribable for disaccharide and/or whole protein intolerance where additional medium chain triglyceride is not indicated. Pepti-Junior, and Pregestimil are ACBS prescribable for disaccharide and/or whole protein intolerance where amino acids or peptides are indicated in conjunction with medium chain triglyceride.								
Indications: suitable for cow's milk intolerance, particularly for infants with gastro-intestinal symptoms. Protein hydrolysate containing MCT, is suitable for infants with fat malabsorption e.g. liver disease or cystic fibrosis.								
Casein hydrolysate								
Nutramigen® (Mead Johnson)	68	283	Casein hydrolysate	1.9	Glucose syrup solids, modified corn starch	7.4	Palm olein oil, coconut oil, soya oil, sunflower oil,	3.4
Pregestimil® (Mead Johnson)	68	283	Casein hydrolysate	1.9	Glucose polymer, modified corn starch, dextrose, maltodextrin	6.9	MCT oil, corn oil, soya oil, safflower oil	3.8
Whey hydrolysate								
Pepti-Junior® (Cow and Gate)	67	280	Whey hydrolysate	1.8	Glucose syrup	6.8	Corn oil, MCT oil, soybean oil, rapeseed oil	3.6

Name of formula	Energy/100mL		Protein	g/100mL	Carbohydrate	g/100mL	Fat	g/100mL
	kcal	KJ						
Soya formula: ACBS listed for proven lactose intolerance in pre-school children, galactokinase deficiency, galactosaemia, and proven whole cow's milk sensitivity.								
Indications: use for infants with cow's milk protein intolerance, galactosaemia, and secondary lactose intolerance.								
Farley's soya formula (HJ Heinz)	70	293	Soya protein isolate	1.9	Glucose syrup	7	Sunflower oil, palm kernal oil, rapeseed oil, palm olein oil	3.8
InfaSoy® (Cow and Gate)	66	275	Soya protein isolate	1.8	Glucose syrup	6.7	Palm oil, sunflower oil rapeseed oil, coconut oil.	3.6
Isomil® (Abbott Nutrition)	68	285	Soya protein isolate	1.8	Corn syrup solids, sucrose	6.9	Sunflower oil, coconut, soya oil	3.7
Prosobee® (Mead Johnson)	68	280	Soya protein isolate	1.8	Glucose polymers	6.7	Palm olein oil, coconut oil, soya oil, sunflower oil	3.7
Wysoy® (SMA Nutrition)	67	280	Soya protein isolate	1.8	Glucose syrup	6.9	Palm oil, coconut oil sunflower oil, soya oil	3.6

Name of formula	Energy/100mL		Protein	g/100mL	Carbohydrate	g/100mL	Fat	g/100mL
	kcal	KJ						
Amino acid formula: ACBS prescribable for disaccharide or dietary protein intolerance in infancy where an elemental formula is specifically indicated.								
Indications: use for severe cow's milk protein intolerance, when protein hydrolysate or soya formula is not tolerated.								
Neocate® (SHS)	71	298	L-amino acids	1.9	Glucose syrup	8.1	Safflower oil, coconut oil, soya oil	3.5

A

Abbreviations *viii*
Abelcet® 28
Accuhaler® 268
Acetazolamide 1
Acetylcysteine (N-acetylcysteine, NAC) 3
Aciclovir (acyclovir) 4
Activated charcoal 8
Acute seizure *xii*
Acyclovir. See Aciclovir
Adenosine 9
Adrenaline (epinephrine) 10
Adverse reactions *x*
Aerochamber® 43, 51, 181, 270
Alfa D® 13
Alfacalcidol (1α-hydroxycholecalciferol) 12
Alimemazine (trimeprazine) tartrate 14
Alpha tocopheryl acetate. See Vitamin E
Ambisome® 28
Amethocaine. See Tetracaine

Ametop® 292
Amikacin 15
Amiloride 18
Aminophylline 19
Amiodarone hydrochloride 21
Amitriptyline 23
Amoxicillin (amoxycillin) 25
Amoxicillin and clavulanic acid. See Co-amoxiclav 91
Amoxycillin. See Amoxicillin
Amphocil® 28
Amphotericin 28
Ampicillin 32
Anaphylaxis *xii*
Aspirin 34
Asthma (acute severe) *xi*
Asystole *xi*
Atenolol 35
Atracurium besilate (besylate) 36
Atropine sulphate 37
Autohaler® 41
Azathioprine 38

Azithromycin 39

B

Babyhaler® 144
Baclofen 40
Beclometasone dipropionate 41
Becodisks® 41
Bendrofluazide. See Bendroflumethiazide
Bendroflumethiazide (bendrofluazide) 43
Benzylpenicillin (penicillin G) 44
Betamethasone esters
    cream, ointment 95
    lotion, foam 95
    scalp application 95
Bisacodyl 46
Bowel cleansing solutions 47
Budesonide 49
Bupivacaine hydrochloride 51

C

Caffeine citrate 52

Calcichew® 53
Calciparine® 163
Calcit® 53
Calcium (oral supplements) 56
Calcium carbonate 53
Calcium chloride 54
Calcium gluconate 55
Calcium Sandoz® 56
Calcium-500® 53
Calculation of body surface area *xiii*
  children and adults *xvi*
  infants *xv*
Canusal® 163
Captopril 58
Carbamazepine 59
Carbimazole 60
Cefaclor 61
Cefadroxil 62
Cefalexin (cephalexin) 63
Cefixime 64

Cefradine (cephradine) 66
Ceftazidime 68
Ceftriaxone 70
Cefuroxime 71
Cephalexin. See Cefalexin
Cephradine. See Cefradine
Chloral hydrate 74
Chloramphenicol 75
Chlorothiazide 78
Chlorphenamine (chlorpheniramine) 80
Chlorpheniramine. See Chlorphenamine
Ciclosporin (cyclosporin) 81
Cimetidine 83
Ciprofloxacin 84
Citramag® 48
Claforan® 66
Clarithromycin 85, 86
Clavulanic acid and amoxicillin 91
Clickhaler® 268
Clindamycin 87, 88

Clobetasol propionate
  cream, ointment 95
  scalp application 95
Clobetasone butyrate
  cream, ointment 95
Clonazepam 89
Co-amoxiclav (amoxicillin and clavulanic acid) 91
Co-trimoxazole 93
Codeine phosphate 94
Corticosteroids (topical) 95
Croup (acute severe) *xi*
Cyclizine 99
Cyclophosphamide 101
Cyclosporin. See Ciclosporin

D

Dalteparin sodium 103
DDAVP® 107
Desmopressin 104
Desmotabs® 106

Diamorphine hydrochloride 111
Diazepam 113
Diazoxide 116
Diclofenac sodium 117
Digoxin 119
Dihydrocodeine tartrate 124
Diocalm Junior® 236
Dioralyte®
   effervescent tablets 236
   relief sachets 236
   sachets 236
Dobutamine hydrochloride 125
Docusate Sodium 126
Domperidone 127
Dopamine hydrochloride 128

E

Electrolade® 236
Emergencies
   acute seizure *xii*
   anaphylaxis *xii*
   asystole *xi*
   hypoglycaemia *xii*
   respiratory *xi*
   shock *xii*
Enalapril 130
Enoxaparin 131
Epinephrine. See Adrenaline
Ergocalciferol (calciferol, vitamin D$_2$) 132
Erythromycin 133
Ethambutol 136
Evohaler® 144

F

Fersamal® 181
Fletcher's enemette® 126
Flucloxacillin 137
Fluconazole 139
Fludrocortisone acetate 141
Flumazenil 142
Fluticasone propionate 143
Folic acid 145

Frusemide. See Furosemide
Fungizone® 28
Furosemide (frusemide) 147
Fusidic acid. See Sodium fusidate

G

Gabapentin 148
Ganciclovir 150
Gaviscon® 153
Gentamicin 154
Glossary of symbols *ix*
Glossary of terms *vii*
Glucagon 158
Glycopyronium bromide 159
Griseofulvin 161

H

Hep-Flush® 163
Heparin 161
Heplok® 163
Humalog® 176, 179

Human Actrapid® 177
Human albumin solution 163
Human Insulatard® 177
Human Mixtard® 178
Human Monotard® 177
Human Ultratard® 178
Human Velosulin® 177
Humulin I® 177
Humulin Lente® 177
Humulin M® 178
Humulin S® 177
Humulin Zn® 178
Hydralazine 164
Hydrocortisone 166
Hydrocortisone cream, ointment 95
Hyoscine hydrobromide 168
Hypnoval® 213
Hypoglycaemia *xii*
Hypostop® 170

I

Immunoglobulin (intravenous) 172
Indometacin (indomethacin) 173
Indomethacin. See Indometacin
InfaSoy® 317
Insulin 175
Insuman® 177, 178
Introductory notes *v*
Ipratropium bromide 180
Iron 181
Isomil® 317
Isoniazid 183
Isoprenaline 184

K

Ketovite® 220
Klean-prep® 48
Konakion® 312

L

Labetalol 185

Levothyroxine (thyroxine) sodium 190
Lidocaine (lignocaine) & prilocaine cream-Emla® 194
Lidocaine (lignocaine) hydrochloride 191
Life support *xi*
Lioresal® 40
Loperamide 196
Lorazepam 197

M

Mannitol 199
Melatonin 200
Meropenem 201
Methylphenidate hydrochloride 203
Methylprednisolone 204
Metoclopramide hydrochloride 205
Metronidazole 207
Midazolam 210
Minims® sodium chloride 274
Monoparin Calcium® 163
Monoparin® 163

Multiparin® 163
Multivitamins 217

N

Naloxone 222
Naproxen 224
Nebuhaler® 51, 181, 292
Nebules® 270
Neocate® 318
Netilmicin 225
Nifedipine 227
Niferex® 181
Nitrazepam 229
Nitrofurantoin 230
Norgalax Micro-enema® 126
NovoMix® 179
NovoRapid® 176
Nutramigen® 316
Nystatin 231

O

Omeprazole 232
Ondansetron 234
One-Alpha® 13
Orakay® 312
Oral Rehydration Salts 236
Ossopan® 56
Osterprem® 182
Ostram® 56
Oxybutynin 237

P

Pancuronium bromide 238
Paracetamol 239
Paraldehyde 242
Penicillin G. See Benzylpenicillin 44
Penicillin V. See Phenoxymethylpenicillin
Pepti-Junior® 316
Pethidine hydrochloride 243
Phenobarbital (phenobarbitone) 244

Phenobarbitone. See Phenobarbital
Phenoxymethylpenicillin (penicillin V) 246
Phenytoin 247
Picolax® 47
Piperacillin with Tazobactam 250
Plesmet® 181
Polyfusor® 272
Potassium chloride 251
Prednisolone 253
Pregestimil® 316
Promethazine hydochloride 257
Propofol 258
Propofol-Lipuro® 259
Propranolol 260
Prosobee® 317
Pump-Hep® 163
Pyridoxine 262

Q

Qvar® 41

R

Ranitidine 264
Rehidrat® 236
Respiratory emergencies *xi*
Respules® 51
Rifampicin 265

S

Salbutamol 268
Salmeterol 270
Sandocal® 56
Scopoderm TTS® 169
Senna 271
Shock *xii*
Sodium bicarbonate 272
Sodium chloride 274
Sodium fusidate/fusidic acid 275
Sodium picosulfate (sodium picosulphate) 277
Sodium picosulphate. See Sodium picosulfate
Sodium valproate 277

Sucralfate 281
Sulfasalazine (sulphasalazine) 282
Sulphamethoxazole and trimethoprim. See
Co-trimoxazole 96
Sulphasalazine. See Sulfasalazine
Sumatriptan 284
Surfactants
    natural 285
    synthetic 286
Sytron® 181

T

Teicoplanin 287
Temazepam 289
Terbutaline 290
Tetracaine (amethocaine) – Ametop® 292
Theophylline 293
Tinzaparin sodium 295
Titralac® 53
Tobramycin 296

Transcop® 169
Trimethoprim 302
Trimethoprim and sulphamethoxazole. See
Co-trimoxazole 96

U

Unihep® 163
Ursodeoxycholic acid 305
Ursofalk® 305

V

Vancomycin 306
Ventodisks® 268
Vigabatrin 309
Vitamin E (Alpha tocopheryl acetate) 310
Vitamin K 312
Volraman® 119
Volumatic® 43, 144, 181, 270

W